Cancer Dissemination Pathways

Daniele Regge, Candiolo Cancer Center,
Torino, Italy   *Series Editor*

This series uses a practical and clinically driven approach to describe the pathways of cancer dissemination, enabling readers to select the best therapeutic option for each patient and to predict disease outcome. Each volume includes an introduction to the morphopathological characteristics and genetic drivers of tumour spread, followed by a chapter describing the radiological signs and pathways of diffusion. The subsequent chapters include a systematic review of pathways of dissemination of each neoplasm. The content is presented schematically, with high-quality illustrations and images obtained from various imaging modalities. The clinical significance of findings and possible therapeutic options is also described where relevant.

More information about this series at http://www.springer.com/series/13608

Daniele Regge
Giulia Zamboni

Editors

Hepatobiliary and Pancreatic Cancer

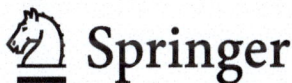

Editors
Daniele Regge
Radiology Unit
University of Torino
Dept. of Surgical Sciences
Candiolo Cancer Center
Candiolo (Torino), Italy

Giulia Zamboni
Institute of Radiology
University Hospital GB Rossi
Verona, Italy

ISSN 2510-3474   ISSN 2510-3482   (electronic)
Cancer Dissemination Pathways
ISBN 978-3-030-09594-9   ISBN 978-3-319-50296-0   (eBook)
https://doi.org/10.1007/978-3-319-50296-0

This Springer imprint is published by Springer Nature
The registered company is Springer International Publishing AG
The registered company address is: Gewerbestrasse 11, 6330 Cham, Switzerland

Foreword

The editors of this book, Prof. Dr. Daniele Regge and Dr. Giulia Zamboni, are highly esteemed experts in the field of abdominal and oncologic imaging. Together with other eminent imaging scientists in this area, they compiled a most informative book. The reader can acquire valuable and practical information on tumors of the hepatobiliary and pancreatic system and the spread of these neoplasms. After an introductory chapter on the principal mechanisms of tumor dissemination, specific hepatobiliary and pancreatic tumor entities, such as hepatocellular carcinoma, cholangiocarcinoma, bile duct and gallbladder tumors, pancreatic adenocarcinoma, neuroendocrine pancreatic tumors, mucinous carcinoma, and IPMN are discussed.

All chapters follow a common structure: after an overview on epidemiology, risk factors, pathology, diagnosis, staging and treatment, and the patterns of local as well as regional and distal spread are described.

I found this book to be a very informative and stimulating read. The presentations are concise and easy to follow for the reader. Understanding is supported by excellent radiological images and illustrated by schematic representations. The pathology and the natural history of the diseases are mentioned so that the dissemination pathways can be reproduced. This also allows for understanding the therapeutic implications of radiological findings and should enable the readers to generate correct and meaningful radiological reports.

In this book, the most recent tumor classifications and guidelines are shown and critically discussed, which again should help the radiologist put his or her findings into perspective and thereby contribute to state-of-the-art therapy planning.

I am indeed convinced that this book may greatly contribute to adequate and precise assessment and treatment planning in patients with hepatobiliary and pancreatic tumors. I hope it will achieve the great success it rightly deserves.

Maximilian Reiser
Department of Radiology
Ludwig-Maximilians-University of Munich
Munich, Germany

Contents

Contributors

Maria Chiara Ambrosetti
UOC Radiologia BR, AOUI Verona
Verona, Italy
mtchiara.ambrosetti@gmail.com

Matilde Bacchion
Dipartimento Chirurgico
Ospedale P. Pederzoli
Verona, Italy
bacchiamat@yahoo.it

Irene Bargellini
Department of Interventional Radiology
Pisa University Hospital
Pisa, Italy
irenebargellini@hotmail.com

Alex Borin
Chirurgia generale e del pancreas
Istituto del Pancreas, AOUI Verona
Verona, Italy
alexborin@live.it

Giovanni Cappello
Department of Surgical Sciences
University of Torino
Torino, Italy

Radiology Unit
Candiolo Cancer Institute – FPO, IRCCS
Candiolo, TO, Italy
giovanni.cappello@ircc.it

Stefano Cavanna
Department of Radiology
Ospedale Mauriziano
Turin, Italy
scavanna@mauriziano.it

Stefano Cirillo
Department of Radiology
Ospedale Mauriziano
Turin, Italy
scirillo@mauriziano.it

Laura Coletti
Department of Liver Surgery and Transplantation
Pisa University Hospital
Pisa, Italy
laura.colettinb@gmail.com

Alessandro Ferrero
Department of General
and Oncological Surgery
Ospedale Mauriziano
Turin, Italy
aferrero@mauriziano.it

Teresa Gallo
Department of Radiology
Ospedale Mauriziano
Turin, Italy
tgallo@mauriziano.it

Giulia Lorenzoni
Department of Interventional Radiology
Pisa University Hospital
Pisa, Italy
lorenzoni.giulia@hotmail.it

Laura Maggino
Chirurgia generale e del pancreas
Istituto del Pancreas, AOUI Verona
Verona, Italy
laura.maggino@hotmail.it

Giuseppe Malleo
Chirurgia generale e del pancreas
Istituto del Pancreas, AOUI Verona
Verona, Italy
giuseppe.malleo@aovr.veneto.it

Giovanni Marchegiani
Chirurgia generale e del pancreas
Istituto del Pancreas, AOUI Verona
Verona, Italy
marcheg@hotmail.it

Marco Miotto
Chirurgia generale e del pancreas
Istituto del Pancreas, AOUI Verona
Verona, Italy
mi8marco@yahoo.it

Roberto Pozzi Mucelli
UOC Radiologia BR, AOUI Verona
Verona, Italy
roberto.pozzimucelli@univr.it

Contributors

Alberto Pisacane
Pathology Unit
Candiolo Cancer Institute – FPO, IRCCS
Candiolo, TO, Italy
alberto.pisacane@ircc.it

Daniele Regge
Department of Surgical Sciences
University of Torino, Candiolo Cancer Center
Candiolo, TO, Italy
daniele.regge@ircc.it

Maxime Ronot
Department of Radiology
University Hospitals Paris Nord Val de Seine
Clichy (Hauts-de-Seine), France

University Paris Diderot
Paris, France

INSERM U1149
Centre de recherche biomédicale
Bichat-Beaujon
Paris, France
maxime.ronot@aphp.fr

Nadia Russolillo
Department of General
and Oncological Surgery
Ospedale Mauriziano
Turin, Italy
nrussolillo@mauriziano.it

Valérie Vilgrain
Department of Radiology,
University Hospitals Paris Nord Val de Seine
Clichy (Hauts-de-Seine), France

University Paris Diderot
Paris, France

INSERM U1149
Centre de recherche biomédicale
Bichat-Beaujon
Paris, France
valerie.vilgrain@bjn.aphp.fr

Giulia Zamboni
UOC Radiologia BR, AOUI Verona
Verona, Italy
giulia.zamboni@aovr.veneto.it

Abbreviations

ADC	Apparent diffusion coefficient	MEN1	Multiple endocrine neoplasia type 1
AFP	Alfa-fetoprotein	MRCP	Magnetic resonance cholangiopancreatography
AJCC	American Joint Committee on Cancer	MRI	Magnetic resonance imaging
		MVI	Microvascular invasion
BCLC	Barcelona Clinic Liver Cancer		
BD-IPMN	Branch duct IPMN	NCAM	Neural cell adhesion molecules
BRPC	Borderline resectable pancreatic cancer	NCCN	National Comprehensive Cancer Network
BTT	Biliary tumor thrombus	NF1	Neurofibromatosis type 1
		NK	Natural Killer
CT	Computed tomography		
cTNM	Clinical tumor-node-metastasis	PC	Plexus pancreaticus capitalis
		PDAC	Pancreatic ductal adenocarcinoma
DWI	Diffusion weighted imaging	PET	Positron emission tomography
		PNET	Pancreatic neuroendocrine tumors
EASL	European Association for the Study of the Liver	PNI	Perineural invasion
ENETS	European Neuroendocrine Tumor Society	PRRT	Peptide receptor radionuclide therapy
eCC	Extrahepatic cholangiocarcinoma	pTNM	Pathological tumor-node-metastasis
ECM	Extracellular matrix		
EM	Extrahepatic metastasis	PTV	Peritumoral lymphatic vessels
		PVE	Portal vein embolization
NAFLD	Nonalcoholic fatty liver disease	PVI	Portal vein vascular invasion
GC	Gallbladder carcinoma	RCT	Randomized controlled trial
GB	Gallbladder	RF	Radiofrequency
		RLN	Regional lymph nodes
HVI	Hepatic vein vascular invasion		
HCC	Hepatocellular carcinoma	SEER	Surveillance, Epidemiology, and End Results
HGDN	High-grade dysplastic nodules	SLN	Sentinel lymph node
HIV	Human immunodeficiency virus	SMV	Superior mesenteric vein
iCC	Intrahepatic cholangiocarcinoma	SSA	Somatostatin analogues
IPMN	Intraductal papillary mucinous neoplasms	TACE	Trans-catheter arterial chemoembolization
IPNB	Intraductal papillary neoplasm of the bile duct	TAE	Trans-catheter arterial embolization
ISGPS	International Study Group of Pancreatic Surgery	TNM	Tumor-node-metastasis
		TSC	Tuberous sclerosis complex
LGDN	Low-grade dysplastic nodules	UICC	Union Internationale Contre le Cancer/International Union Against Cancer
LI-RADS	Liver Imaging Reporting and Data System		
LTx	Liver transplantation	US	Ultrasound
MCN	Mucinous cystic neoplasms	VHL	von Hippel Lindau
MDCT	Multidetector computer tomography	WHO	World Health Organization
MD-IPMN	Main duct IPMN	Y90-RE	Yttrium-90 labeled spheres

Mechanism of Tumour Dissemination in Hepatobiliary and Pancreatic Tumours

Daniele Regge, Giovanni Cappello, and Alberto Pisacane

© Springer International Publishing AG 2018
D. Regge, G. Zamboni (eds.), *Hepatobiliary and Pancreatic Cancer*,
Cancer Dissemination Pathways, https://doi.org/10.1007/978-3-319-50296-0_1

1

1.1 Local Spread

Local spread is defined as the diffusion of a tumour within an organ or throughout adjacent structures by contiguity. It represents the ability of cancer cells to thrust aside adjacent tissues to actively invade them and/or destroy them [1]. Tumours may either expand into adjacent tissues, spread locally through direct infiltration or disseminate along blood and lymphatic vessels, nerves, and excretory biliary ducts.

1.1.1 Expansive Growth

Location and tumour characteristics affect the ability of cancer cells to spread locally. Some tumours, such as hepatocellular carcinoma (HCC), may have an inclination for *expansive growth*. Compression of the liver parenchyma by the expanding tumour may stimulate the development of a capsule that is composed of an inner layer of tight relatively pure fibrous tissue containing thin slit like vascular channels, and of an outer layer composed of looser fibrovascular tissue containing portal venules, bile ducts, and prominent sinusoids [2, 3] (◉ Fig. 1.1). Patients

with intact tumour capsule have a higher survival rate, suggesting that the capsule is a physical barrier to tumour spread [3–5].

Expansive growth is common also in intrahepatic cholangiocarcinoma (iCC) where malignant cells penetrate the bile duct wall and spread between the hepatocyte layers infiltrating the hepatic sinusoidal spaces [6]. Surrounded by liver parenchyma, iCC grows three-dimensionally, presenting itself as an irregularly but well-defined shaped solid mass [7, 8], not invading a major branch of the portal triad and with a peripheral fibrous component [7, 9]. iCC is rarely symptomatic in the early stages [6] and can achieve a large dimension before being diagnosed. Patients may develop symptoms when the large mass causes compression and dilatation of a large bile duct or when liver capsular invasion and retraction is present.

Pancreatic mucinous cystic neoplasms (MCN) are frequently characterized by an expansive growth. Typically, they appear as thick walled, unilocular/multilocular cystic tumours [10] surrounded by a capsule composed of an inner epithelial layer secreting mucin and by an external layer of dense cellular ovarian-type stroma [11]. In a late phase, invasive carcinoma cells may infiltrate the capsule and reach its outer layer (intracapsular invasion) or

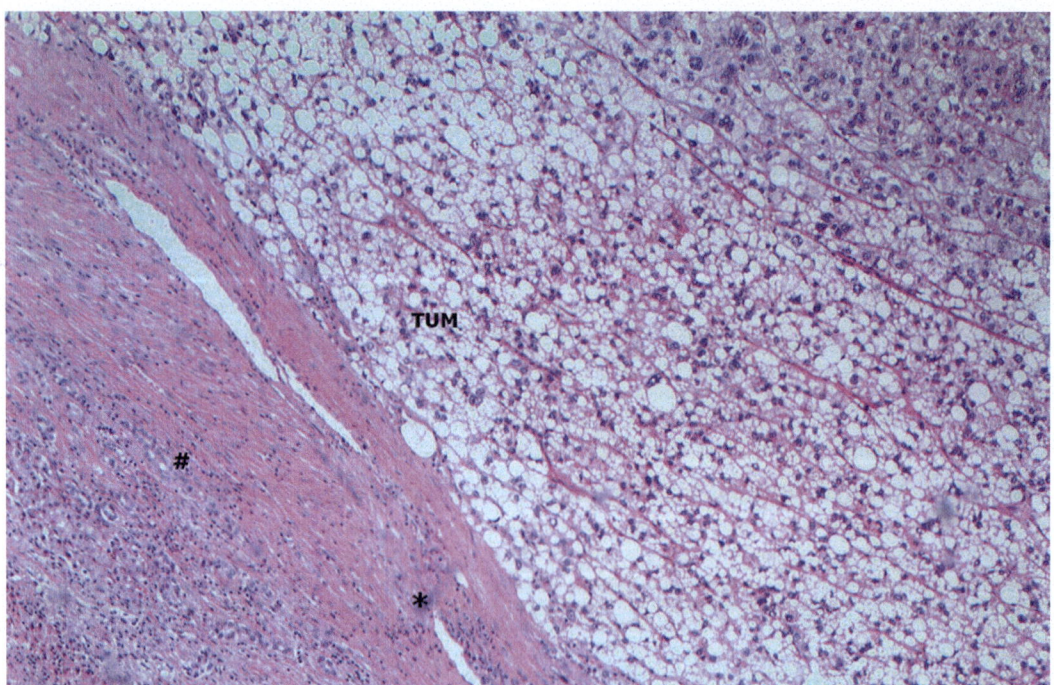

◉ Fig. 1.1   Tumour capsule in HCC (*Tum*); inner layer with slit like vascular channels (*asterisk*) and outer layer (*hash*)

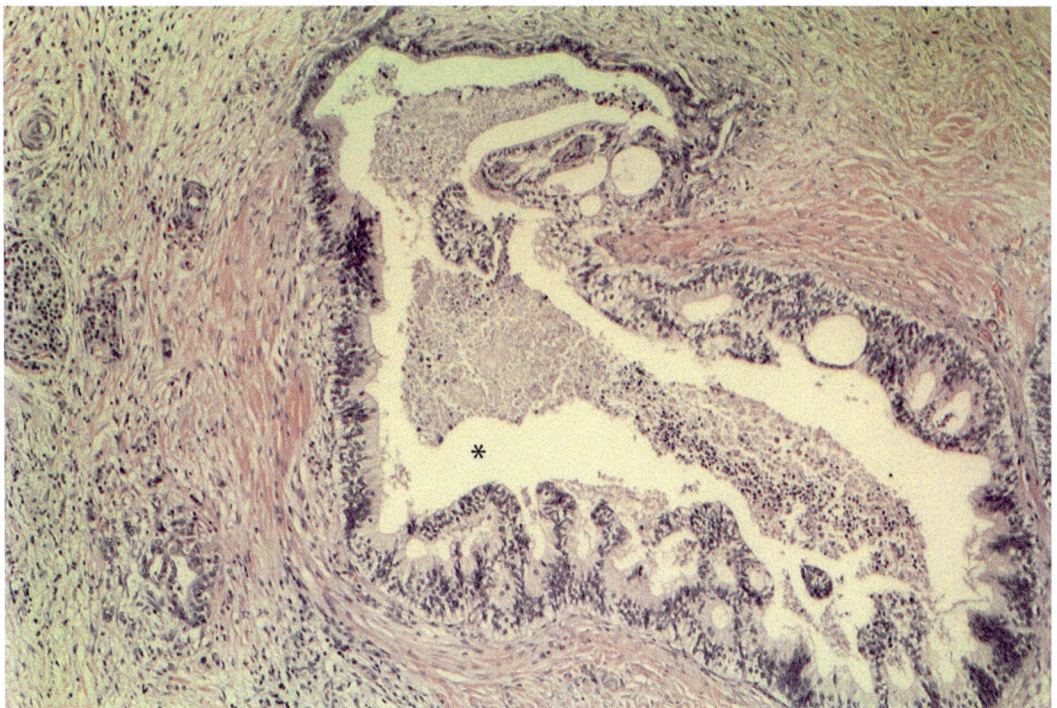

◘ Fig. 1.2 Extrahepatic cholangiocarcinoma; intraductal growth in a dilated bile duct (*asterisk*)

extend into the surrounding pancreatic tissue and/or thrust within the peritoneal cavity (extracapsular invasion) [12]. Spread of tumour through vascular, lymphatic, or neural structures is however a rare occurrence and this partly explains the favourable prognosis of MCN in comparison to the more aggressive pancreatic adenocarcinoma [10].

Extrahepatic cholangiocarcinoma (eCC) may extend to the bile duct or gallbladder wall by either intraductal, nodular or infiltrative growth [13, 14]. The intraductal eCC type has a distinct expansive growth pattern that can be characterized by a superficial mucosal spread along the bile duct lumen [6, 13, 15] (reported in 10–75% of cases) [13]. It can form intraductal papilla or mime a tumour thrombus, leading to peripheral bile duct dilatation (◘ Fig. 1.2). Extension through the duct wall and stromal invasion is rare and explains the better prognosis of this type of eCC [14, 15].

1.1.2 Infiltrative Growth

Most pancreatic and biliary tumours have an infiltrative behaviour, which partly explains their dismal prognosis. From a pathological standpoint two different intramural infiltration growth-types

have been observed in gallbladder cancer: the infiltrative growth-type, with muscle preservation, and the destructive growth-type where the muscle layer is destroyed [16–18]. The latter generally presents a more aggressive behaviour, also leading to a higher probability of lympho-vascular spread [16–18].

The aggressive behaviour of some tumours has also been linked to their surrounding environment. In pancreatic ductal cancer, for example, tumour–stromal interactions contribute in oncogenic signalling, promoting the synthetization of different components of the extracellular matrix (ECM), which stimulate the formation of a marked fibrosis and dense desmoplastic reaction, leading to a fibroblast-mediated tumour growth and progression [19–21]. Macroscopically, pancreatic adenocarcinoma forms a solid and firm, highly sclerotic mass, with poorly defined tumour burden and sends long tongues of neoplastic cells extending beyond the main tumour [22, 23] (◘ Fig. 1.3). Because the pancreas is not enclosed in a distinct capsule, the tumour easily invades the surrounding pancreatic fatty tissue, resulting in an infiltration of the prosperous network of lymphatic, vascular, and nerve structures and in a dissemination of

1

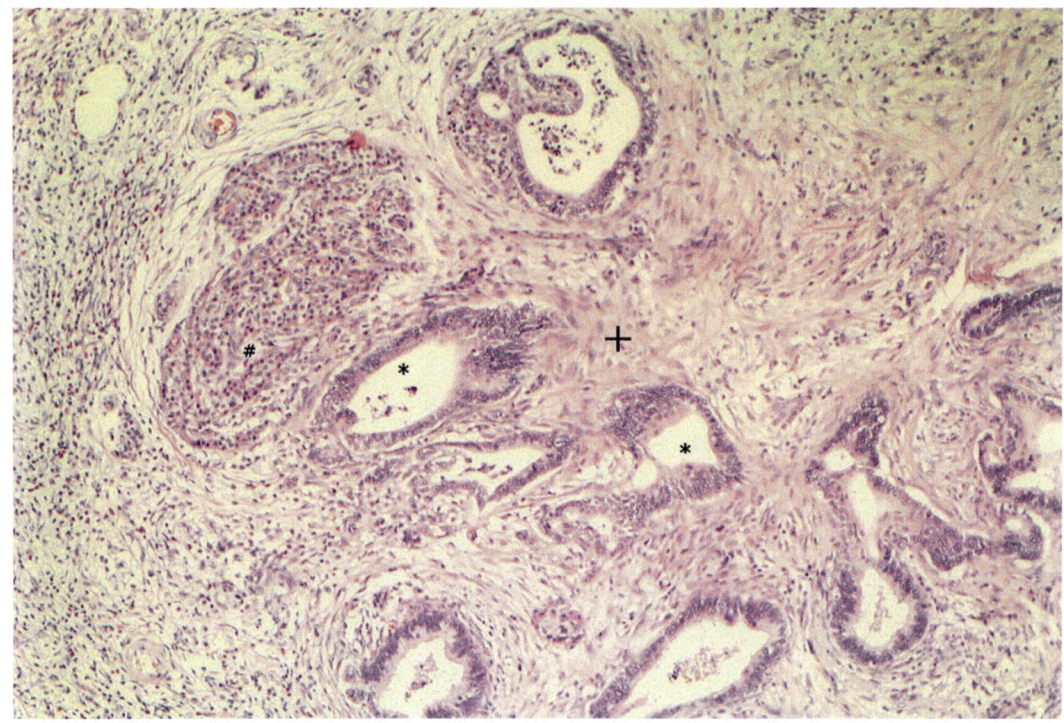

▢ Fig. 1.3 Infiltrative growth in pancreatic adenocarcinoma; tongues of neoplastic glandular tissue (*asterisk*) in a reactive, desmoplastic stroma (*plus*) infiltrating through involuted pancreatic parenchyma (*hash*)

malignant cells throughout these routes [23]. The pancreas is located in the retroperitoneal space and presents a very close anatomic relationship with a broad variety of structures and organs in the upper abdomen [24]. As a result, by the time it is detected pancreatic adenocarcinoma has usually spread beyond the gland invading adjacent organs by contiguity. Tumours arising from the pancreatic head or uncinated process are often associated with a direct compression or invasion of the bile duct and the duodenum while tumours originating from the body or the tail may directly involve the stomach and spleen [25, 26].

Infiltrative spread is influenced by the anatomy of the organ where the tumour originates. The gallbladder wall, for example, is composed of only four layers: mucosa, lamina propria, an irregular muscle layer, and externally by a thin stratum of connective tissue [18, 27, 28]. The absence of the submucosal layer and the irregular presence of the muscular layer make it easy for the tumour to cross the GB wall and to invade the adjacent structures by contiguity [27–30]. Moreover, since the hepatic surface of the GB lacks of the serosa layer, the connective tissue of the GB is continuous

with the interlobular connective tissue of the liver. These unique anatomical characteristics explain why the direct infiltration of the liver and of the sub-hepatic space are the most common routes of local dissemination in GB cancer originating from the fundus or body [18, 28]. Conversely, tumours arising from the GB neck spread along the cystic duct and reach the extrahepatic bile duct, resulting in biliary obstruction [28, 31].

1.2 Metastases

Metastases arise from the spread of cancer from the primary site to distant organs. The metastatic process consists of a series of steps all of which must be accomplished for metastatic tumour to develop (▢ Scheme 1.1). When the primary tumour reaches a size of 1–2 mm new vessels develop to provide nutrients and oxygen to cancer cells. These vessels also allow cancer cells to migrate through the endothelial barrier into the blood stream. Cells that survive in the blood circulation may extravasate in a new organ and enter the surrounding tissue where they can grow and develop new blood vessels. Tumour may spread to distant organs also

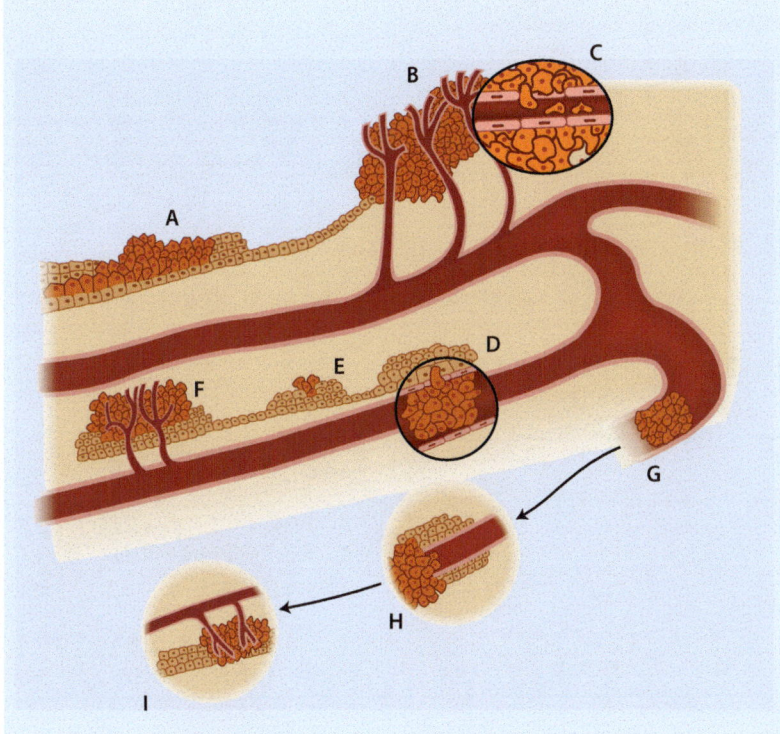

■ **Scheme 1.1** Steps of the metastatic cascade. During tumour growth (*A*), an increased amount of nutrients and oxygen is required by cancer cells. For this reason, the tumour produces growth factors, which stimulate the formation of new vessels (neoangiogenesis) (*B*). The highly permeable newly formed capillaries favour the migration of cancer cells into the blood stream where they can spread to other tissues (circulation) (*C*). Because of their dimensions, malignant cells get stuck in the lumen of capillaries where they proliferate forming an intraluminal thrombus and then extravasate (*D*). Once in the new site, cancer cells may remain dormant for a long time (*E*) or they may start to grow again, forming a metastasis (*F*). Alternately, the intraluminal thrombus formed by cancer cells (*G*) may grow and determine the destruction of cell walls (*H*) facilitating the access of the proliferating tumour into the new tissue (*I*)

via the lymphatic system. The above described represents a stepwise process that will be explained in more detail in the following sections.

1.2.1 Intravasation

Intravasation refers to the process in which cancer cells enter the lumen of blood vessels or lymphatics [1]. As aforementioned, the uncontrolled growth of cancer cells amplifies the metabolic activity of newly formed tissues which in turn increases the need for nutrients and oxygen. To provide nutrients and oxygen, neoplastic cells secrete growth factors that attract endothelial cells to the tumour; the latter secretes enzymes to degrade the basement line of capillaries and promote the formation of new blood vessels and lymphatics [32–35].

1.2.1.1 Angiogenesis

The process by which tumour neovessels sprout from existing blood vessels is referred to as *tumour angiogenesis* [36]. Tumour vessels are malformed and highly permeable and favour the migration of neoplastic cell into the body blood stream. Characteristically, epithelial cells that give rise to most pancreatic and hepatobiliary cancers are characterized by the absence of motility due to tight cell–cell adhesion and the anchoring to the ECM by the basement membrane [1]. Reorganization of matrix constituents during tumour growth results in the disruption of the architecture of the ECM, promoting cell transformation, tumour cell motility, and migration [37]. Once near a vessel, the proteases produced by the malignant cells degrade the endothelium of the vessel enabling the access of cells into the blood stream [1].

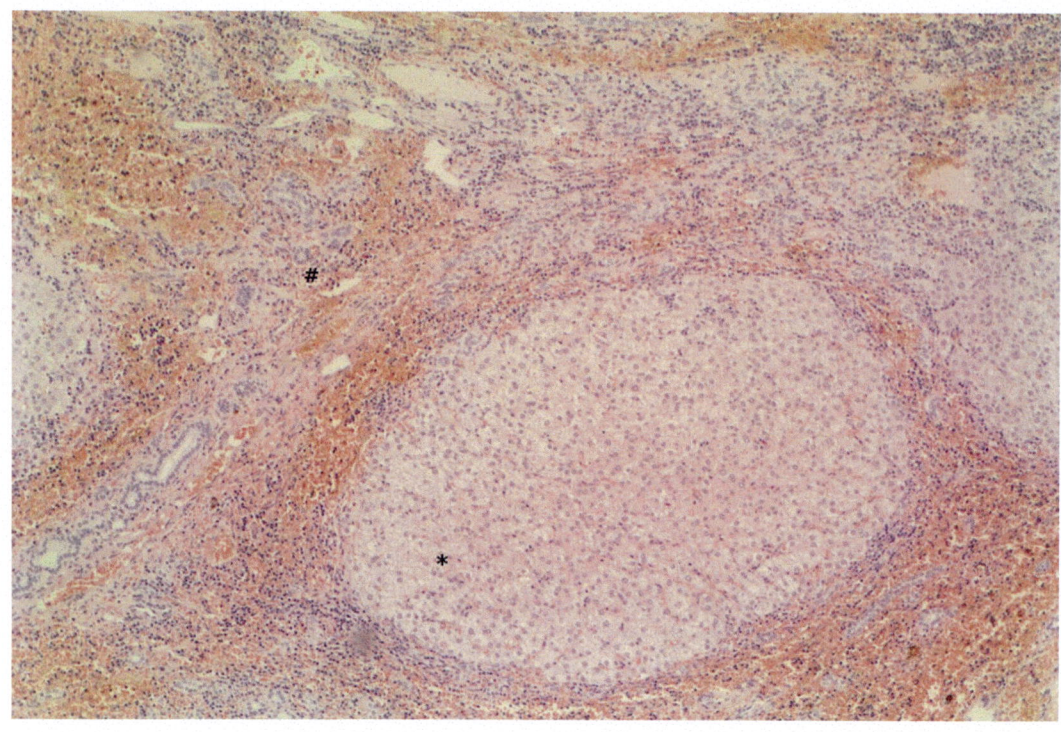

Fig. 1.4   Small satellite nodule of HCC (*asterisk*) and surrounding liver (*hash*)

In HCC, the process of intravasation is akin to the pathological concept of microvascular or macrovascular invasion of blood vessels [3]. Microvascular invasion (MVI) is defined as the presence of microscopic tumour invasion within the small vessels surrounding the tumour edge, visible only at microscopy [38]. Its presence is an important risk factor and determines an increased tumour recurrence rate after surgery [3, 39, 40]. Sumie et al. reported a 3-year recurrence-free survival rate in individuals with HCC that underwent liver resection with and without venous MVI, respectively, of 27.7% and 62.5% [41]. MVI can be mild, when one to five vessels are invaded, or severe, when more than five vessels are invaded [41]. Patients with HCC and severe MVI have a more dismal prognosis [41]. In both HCC and iCC, MVI may involve small veins on the tumour edge and result in the formation of "satellite" nodules within the venous drainage area surrounding the main lesion (▢ Fig. 1.4). Differently from "satellite" nodules, tumour nodules that develop in other liver segments are classified as distant metastases [3].

Macroscopic invasion takes place when the tumour thrombus is visible at gross pathologic examination and/or at imaging [38]. HCC patients with macrovascular invasion have a poor prognosis and surgical resection is usually not a treatment option [42]. It follows that identification of venous invasion at imaging is of paramount importance to plan treatment of these patients and is included in the scoring systems that determine treatment strategies in HCC patients [43–45]. While vascular invasion is exceptional in other types of liver tumours, it may occasionally be observed in pancreatic endocrine tumours [46].

1.2.1.2 Lymphangiogenesis

Lymphatic vessels compass a unidirectional fluid recycling system and play a pivotal role in tumour dissemination [47]. In normal conditions, fluid and cells are uptaken by lymphatic capillaries and conveyed down the lymphatic ducts to the regional lymph nodes and ultimately through the thoracic duct into the venous system [48]. Tumour cells can bolster lymphangiogenesis by altering the surrounding microenvironment and by promoting the secretion of soluble molecules that stimulate the enlargement of tumour lymphatic vessels [49]. Differently from angiogenesis, lymphatic capillaries grow mainly around the tumour (peri-tumoural lymphatic vessels; PTV) while intra-tumoural lymphatic vessels are small,

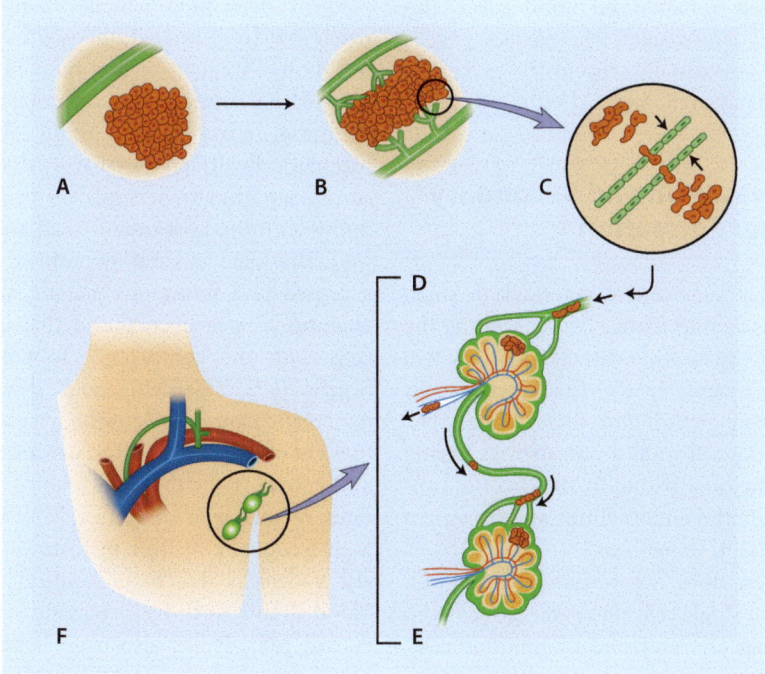

■ **Scheme 1.2** Lymphangiogenesis and lymphatic spread. During tumour growth (*A*), cancer cells secrete lymphangiogenic cytokines which stimulate the growth of new lymphatic vessels, mainly at the tumour edge (*B*). Tumour cells invade the extracellular matrix and infiltrate the lymphatic capillaries (*C*). Malignant cells move with the lymphatic stream into the sentinel lymph node and invade their cortex (*D*). From there, cancer cells can either travel in the lymph, reaching downhill lymph nodes (*E*) and eventually the thoracic duct from where they enter the blood circulation, or intravasate in the blood capillaries of the lymph node (*F*)

collapsed, and non-functional. As a consequence, only the PTV have the capacity to absorb fluid and cells and act as routes for cancer spread to regional lymph nodes [50]. Cancer cells are transported from the tumour to the lymphatic capillaries where the interstitial fluid pressure is lower and invade into their lumen through the open interendothelial gaps [51]. Lymphatic endothelial cells can support the process by secreting chemotactic factors that attract malignant tumour cells within the lymphatic lumen [52].

Tumour cells that enter the lymphatic system are transported to the regional lymph nodes (RLN) and grow to become secondary tumours (■ Scheme 1.2). The first RLN where tumour cells metastasize is the sentinel lymph node (SLN) [53]. From there cancer cells can either travel in the lymph and eventually enter the circulation, or intravasate into the blood capillaries of the lymph node [48, 51]. Most advanced hepatobiliary and pancreatic tumours metastasize to RLN while those in the early stages rarely disseminate into the lymphatic system. In epithelial tumours,

the presence of metastasis in RLN is one of the most important negative prognostic factors. Furthermore, the concept of SLN has dramatically changed the surgical approach to treatment of some tumours, which has evolved in nature from radical to minimal [54].

1.2.2 Circulation

Cancer cells that enter the lumen of vessels or lymphatics migrate to distant tissues and form metastases in other organs. This is an extremely inefficient process as only <0.01% of tumour cells eventually form distant metastases [55, 56]. Typically, a 1-g tumour is composed of billions of cells that can shed 1–4 million cancer cells and most of these will die in the first 24 h by either attrition or direct cytotoxicity and lysis by Natural Killer (NK) cells on immunosurveillance [57]. Liver and lung are very efficient in arresting cancer cells, essentially by size restriction. Liver capillaries are small (3–8 μm in diameter) and are

1

designed to allow transit of red blood cells (7 µm in diameter and deformable), whereas cancer cells are quite large and usually stop in the pre-capillary vessels (20 µm in diameter) [58].

1.2.3 Extravasation and Secondary Tumour Formation

Cancer cells that survive and get stuck in small vessels *extravasate* into tissues by penetrating the endothelium. Extravasation can take place by two different mechanisms. In the first, cancer cells start proliferating within the vessel lumen [1]. With growth, the cell walls are destroyed paving the access to the host tissue. In the second, cancer cells degrade the endothelium and basement membrane through proteolysis [1].

Extravasation does not necessarily result in metastasis. Most single cells that enter tissues from circulation either are destroyed by immune cells, go into apoptose or remain dormant [59]. Some metastases can reside within the new environment without proliferating due to the absence of growth factors of the original tissue [60]. Micro-metastases can undergo various mutations during time, giving the tumour the potential to proliferate. Once the tumour has reached a size of 1–2 mm, neo-angiogenesis takes place regulating the transition between the avascular to the vascular phase [1]. At this point, the patient faces a poor prognosis.

1.2.4 Organ Specificity of Metastases

Metastases show an organ-specific pattern of spread. For example, colorectal cancer has a propensity to metastasize to the liver while breast cancer develops brain, bone, and lung metastases. As mentioned above, other tumours metastasize to RLN and can then either enter blood circulation or keep on travelling in the lymphatic system [47]. Stephen Paget in his 1889 paper [61] observed that "distribution of secondary growths (metastases) was not a matter of chance" and hypothesized the "seed and soil" theory. According to Paget's theory, organ-specific distribution of metastases depended both on the characteristics of cancer cells (the seed) and of the secondary organ (soil). The "seed and soil" theory was later challenged by James Ewing which suggested that blood-flow

patterns determine which organ tumour cells reach first [62]. Indeed, the two mechanisms are not mutually exclusive and probably both have a role in the development of metastases [63–65]: the initial delivery of the tumour cells seems to be mechanically driven (circulatory theory) while the secondary growth depends on tumour compatibility with the host organ (seed and soil theory) [66]. The "seed and soil" hypothesis is now widely accepted and numerous genetic and epigenetic alterations have been found that endow cancer cells with the competence to colonize distant organs [67]. Haematogenous dissemination of pancreatic cancer cells to the liver and the development of aggressive metastases are very common and accounts for the high relapse and mortality rates of this type of cancer [67]. Certainly, the high frequency of liver metastases from pancreatic cancer is due to anatomical reasons since blood drains to the pancreas through the portal system [68]. It has also been hypothesized that blood entering the portal circulation follows a streamline phenomenon such that patients with carcinoma of the tail and body of the pancreas, particularly in the presence of splenic vein invasion, develop metastases preferably in the left lobe [68]. However, the presence of a short latency in metastasis relapse and the aggressiveness of pancreatic adenocarcinoma can be explained only by genetic mechanisms [69]. Like pancreatic adenocarcinoma, diffuse type HCC develops via intrahepatic dissemination of cancer cells through the portal vein in a short period of time [70].

1.3 Perineural Invasion

As described in the previous sections, solid tumours spread in three classical pathways: local tumour spread, lymphatic and vascular dissemination. A fourth, less known route of tumour spread is represented by perineural invasion (PNI) [71]. PNI refers to the process of neoplastic invasion in, around, and through nerves (◘ Scheme 1.3) [72]. This route of dissemination was described for the first time in 1835 by Jean Cruveilheir, a French pathologist, who observed PNI in head and neck tumours [73].

From a pathological perspective, different growth patterns have been described, from a simple abutment on nerve structures to various grade of encasement of the nerve sheath (◘ Fig. 1.5).

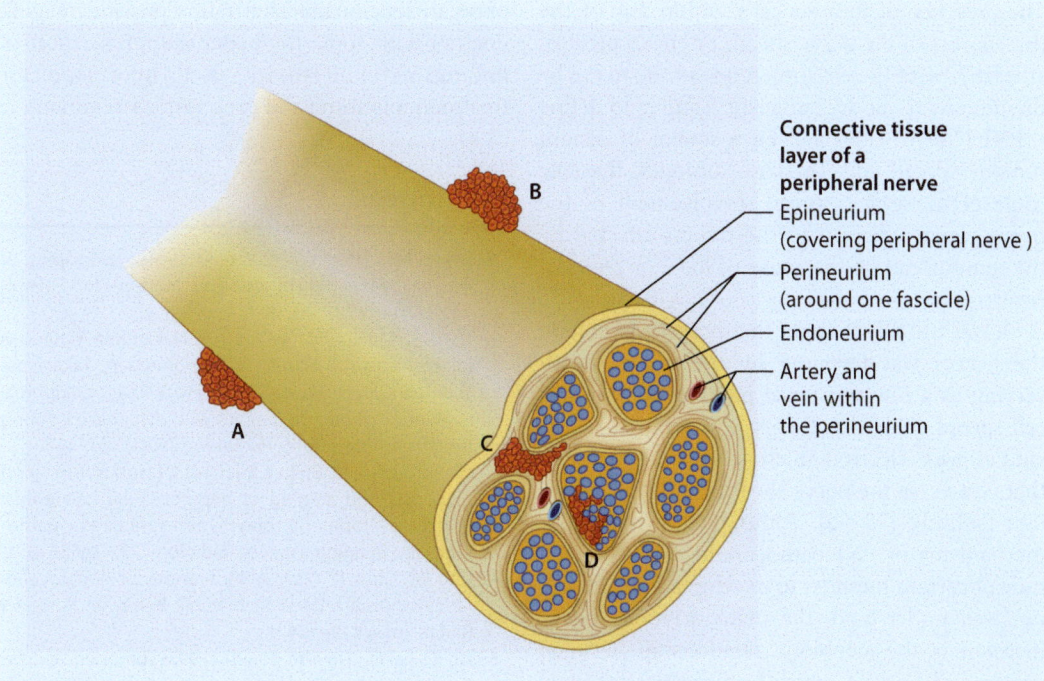

Connective tissue
layer of a
peripheral nerve
Epineurium
(covering peripheral nerve)
Perineurium
(around one fascicle)
Endoneurium
Artery and
vein within
the perineurium

■ **Scheme 1.3**   Perineural invasion. Perineural invasion refers to the process of neoplastic invasion in, around, and through the nerves. A nerve sheath is composed of three tissue layers (from outside in): the epineurium, the perineurium, and the endoneurium. Nerve involvement may be characterized by a simple abutment **a** or infiltration **b** of the epineurium or by the presence of neoplastic cells within the perineurium **c** or in the endoneurium **d**

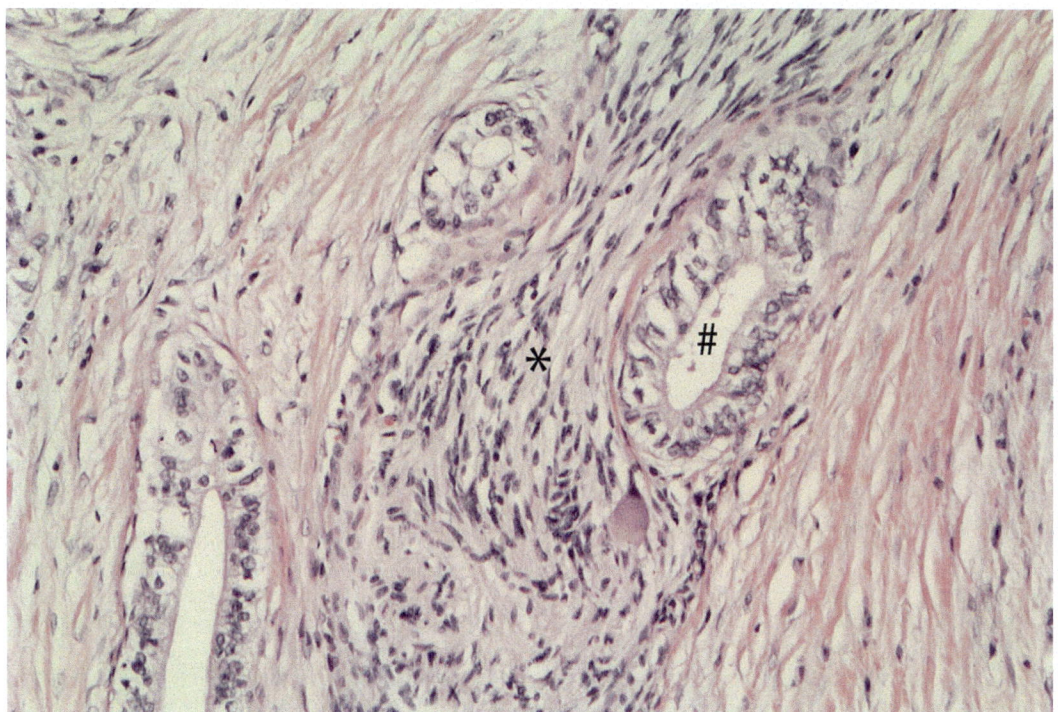

■ **Fig. 1.5**   Perineural invasion (*asterisk*: nerve; *hash*: perineural neoplastic gland)

1

The presence of tumour cells within any of the three layers of the nerve sheath or encasement of at least 33% of the circumference of the nerve by the tumour tissue are sufficient features to define a PNI [74–76]. PNI can be a source of distant tumour spread and, in some tumours, the sole route of metastatic spread. Involvement of the nerve plexus adjacent to the organs affected by the tumour can be the cause of local or regional recurrence.

It was initially thought that progression along the nerves was favoured by the nerve sheath serving as a low resistance pathway for tumour cell spread [77]. This theory was rebutted when studies with electron microscopy demonstrated that vice versa the nerve sheath is a highly resistant pathway [78–80]. Although the molecular mechanisms of PNI pathogenesis and the aptitude of certain tumours to develop a PNI are still not well understood, the main driver of nerve invasion is the symbiotic relationship between cancer and host, in which both parties facilitate the metastatic process [71, 81]. Signalling mechanisms involving tumour cells, nerve cells, and the stromal environment play a pivotal role, through the production of neurotrophins, chemokines, and proteinases, as matrix metalloproteinases, facilitating tumour invasion [82, 83].

In many hepatobiliary malignancies, PNI has emerged as a key pathological feature and a marker of poor disease outcome [82]. PNI is a common finding in pancreatic cancer (70–100% of cases), bile duct cancer (75–85% of cases), and gallbladder carcinoma (44–72% of cases) [82, 84]. In pancreatic cancer, tumour cells extend by PNI through the plexuses from the celiac and superior mesenteric artery ganglia. In such occurrence, complete tumour removal with safe margins is difficult to achieve and is an important determinant of the patient prognosis. In a series of 72 patients with pancreatic cancer and lymph node negative disease, Ozaky et al. [85] reported a 5-year survival rate of 75% in patients without PNI versus 29% in those with PNI.

1.4 Conclusions

Mechanisms of cancer spread have not yet been fully investigated and much still remains to be unveiled. However, current knowledge on the pathways of tumour dissemination and principles of organ-specific metastatization provide imaging doctors with tools for better comprehension of findings and clinicians with useful information for treatment planning and prognostic assessment.

References

1. Leber MF, Efferth T (2009) Molecular principles of cancer invasion and metastasis (review). Int J Oncol 34(4):881–895
2. Ueda K, Matsui O, Kawamori Y, Nakanuma Y, Kadoya M, Yoshikawa J, Gabata T, Nonomura A, Takashima T (1998) Hypervascular hepatocellular carcinoma: evaluation of hemodynamics with dynamic CT during hepatic arteriography. Radiology 206(1):161–166
3. Choi JY, Lee JM, Sirlin CB (2014) CT and MR imaging diagnosis and staging of hepatocellular carcinoma: part I. Development, growth, and spread: key pathologic and imaging aspects. Radiology 272(3):635–654
4. Cho ES, Choi JY (2015) MRI features of hepatocellular carcinoma related to biologic behavior. Korean J Radiol 16(3):449–464
5. Ng IO, Lai EC, Ng MM, Fan ST (1992) Tumor encapsulation in hepatocellular carcinoma. A pathologic study of 189 cases. Cancer 70(1):45–49
6. Lim JH (2003) Cholangiocarcinoma: morphologic classification according to growth pattern and imaging findings. AJR Am J Roentgenol 181(3):819–827
7. Yamasaki S (2003) Intrahepatic cholangiocarcinoma: macroscopic type and stage classification. J Hepatobiliary Pancreat Surg 10(4):288–291
8. Chung YE, Kim MJ, Park YN, Choi JY, Pyo JY, Kim YC, Cho HJ, Kim KA, Choi SY (2009) Varying appearances of cholangiocarcinoma: radiologic-pathologic correlation. Radiographics 29(3):683–700
9. Blechacz B, Komuta M, Roskams T, Gores GJ (2011) Clinical diagnosis and staging of cholangiocarcinoma. Nat Rev Gastroenterol Hepatol 8(9):512–522
10. Fritz S, Warshaw AL, Thayer SP (2009) Management of mucin-producing cystic neoplasms of the pancreas. Oncologist 14(2):125–136
11. Matthaei H, Schulick RD, Hruban RH, Maitra A (2011) Cystic precursors to invasive pancreatic cancer. Nat Rev Gastroenterol Hepatol 8(3):141–150
12. Crippa S, Salvia R, Warshaw AL, Domínguez I, Bassi C, Falconi M, Thayer SP, Zamboni G, Lauwers GY, Mino-Kenudson M, Capelli P, Pederzoli P, Castillo CF (2008) Mucinous cystic neoplasm of the pancreas is not an aggressive entity: lessons from 163 resected patients. Ann Surg 247(4):571–579
13. Nakanishi Y, Zen Y, Kawakami H, Kubota K, Itoh T, Hirano S, Tanaka E, Nakanuma Y, Kondo S (2008) Extrahepatic bile duct carcinoma with extensive intraepithelial spread: a clinicopathological study of 21 cases. Mod Pathol 21(7):807–816
14. Suarez-Munoz MA, Fernandez-Aguilar JL, Sanchez-Perez B, Perez-Daga JA, Garcia-Albiach B, Pulido-Roa Y, Marin-Camero N, Santoyo-Santoyo J (2013) Risk factors and classifications of hilar cholangiocarcinoma. World J Gastrointest Oncol 5(7):132–138

15. Chung YE, Kim MJ, Park YN, Lee YH, Choi JY (2008) Staging of extrahepatic cholangiocarcinoma. Eur Radiol 18(10):2182–2195
16. Okada K, Kijima H, Imaizumi T, Hirabayashi K, Matsuyama M, Yazawa N, Oida Y, Dowaki S, Tobita K, Ohtani Y, Tanaka M, Inokuchi S, Makuuchi H (2009) Wall-invasion pattern correlates with survival of patients with gallbladder adenocarcinoma. Anticancer Res 29(2):685–691
17. Kijima H, Wu Y, Yosizawa T, Suzuki T, Tsugeno Y, Haga T, Seino H, Morohashi S, Hakamada K (2014) Pathological characteristics of early to advanced gallbladder carcinoma and extrahepatic cholangiocarcinoma. J Hepatobiliary Pancreat Sci 21(7):453–458
18. Kanthan R, Senger JL, Ahmed S, Kanthan SC (2015) Gallbladder cancer in the 21st century. J Oncol 2015:967472
19. Mihaljevic AL, Michalski CW, Friess H, Kleeff J (2010) Molecular mechanism of pancreatic cancer–understanding proliferation, invasion, and metastasis. Langenbecks Arch Surg 395(4):295–308
20. Vincent A, Herman J, Schulick R, Hruban RH, Goggins M (2011) Pancreatic cancer. Lancet 378(9791):607–620
21. Korc M (2007) Pancreatic cancer-associated stroma production. Am J Surg 194(4 Suppl):S84–S86
22. Maitra A, Hruban RH (2008) Pancreatic cancer. Annu Rev Pathol 3:157–188
23. Wolfgang CL, Herman JM, Laheru DA, Klein AP, Erdek MA, Fishman EK, Hruban RH (2013) Recent progress in pancreatic cancer. CA Cancer J Clin 63(5):318–348
24. Vikram R, Balachandran A, Bhosale PR, Tamm EP, Marcal LP, Charnsangavej C (2009) Pancreas: peritoneal reflections, ligamentous connections, and pathways of disease spread. Radiographics 29(2):e34
25. Schima W, Ba-Ssalamah A, Kölblinger C, Kulinna-Cosentini C, Puespoek A, Götzinger P (2007) Pancreatic adenocarcinoma. Eur Radiol 17(3):638–649
26. Padilla-Thornton AE, Willmann JK, Jeffrey RB (2012) Adenocarcinoma of the uncinate process of the pancreas: MDCT patterns of local invasion and clinical features at presentation. Eur Radiol 22(5):1067–1074
27. Hussain HM, Little MD, Wei S (2013) AIRP best cases in radiologic-pathologic correlation: gallbladder carcinoma with direct invasion of the liver. Radiographics 33(1):103–108
28. Levy AD, Murakata LA, Rohrmann CA Jr (2001) Gallbladder carcinoma: radiologic-pathologic correlation. Radiographics 21(2):295–314
29. Yoshimitsu K, Honda H, Shinozaki K, Aibe H, Kuroiwa T, Irie H, Chijiiwa K, Asayama Y, Masuda K (2002) Helical CT of the local spread of carcinoma of the gallbladder: evaluation according to the TNM system in patients who underwent surgical resection. AJR Am J Roentgenol 179(2):423–428
30. Wistuba II, Gazdar AF (2004) Gallbladder cancer: lessons from a rare tumour. Nat Rev Cancer 4(9):695–706
31. Lane J, Buck JL, Zeman RK (1989) Primary carcinoma of the gallbladder: a pictorial essay. Radiographics 9(2):209–228
32. Klagsbrun M, D'Amore PA (1991) Regulators of angiogenesis. Annu Rev Physiol 53:217–239
33. Folkman J (1992) The role of angiogenesis in tumor growth. Semin Cancer Biol 3(2):65–71
34. Iruela-Arispe ML, Dvorak HF (1997) Angiogenesis: a dynamic balance of stimulators and inhibitors. Thromb Haemost 78(1):672–677
35. Fidler IJ, Kumar R, Bielenberg DR, Ellis LM (1998) Molecular determinants of angiogenesis in cancer metastasis. Cancer J Sci Am 4(Suppl 1):S58–S66
36. Folkman J (1971) Tumor angiogenesis: therapeutic implications. N Engl J Med 285(21):1182–1186
37. Paduch R (2016) The role of lymphangiogenesis and angiogenesis in tumor metastasis. Cell Oncol (Dordr) 39(5):397–410
38. Pomfret EA, Washburn K, Wald C, Nalesnik MA, Douglas D, Russo M, Roberts J, Reich DJ, Schwartz ME, Mieles L, Lee FT, Florman S, Yao F, Harper A, Edwards E, Freeman R, Lake J (2010) Report of a national conference on liver allocation in patients with hepatocellular carcinoma in the United States. Liver Transpl 16(3):262–278
39. Ünal E, İdilman İS, Akata D, Özmen MN, Karçaaltıncaba M (2016) Microvascular invasion in hepatocellular carcinoma. Diagn Interv Radiol 22(2):125–132
40. Lim JH, Choi D, Park CK, Lee WJ, Lim HK (2006) Encapsulated hepatocellular carcinoma: CT-pathologic correlations. Eur Radiol 16(10):2326–2333
41. Sumie S, Nakashima O, Okuda K, Kuromatsu R, Kawaguchi A, Nakano M, Satani M, Yamada S, Okamura S, Hori M, Kakuma T, Torimura T, Sata M (2014) The significance of classifying microvascular invasion in patients with hepatocellular carcinoma. Ann Surg Oncol 21(3):1002–1009
42. Llovet JM, Fuster J, Bruix J, Barcelona-Clínic Liver Cancer Group (2004) The Barcelona approach: diagnosis, staging, and treatment of hepatocellular carcinoma. Liver Transpl 10(2 Suppl 1):S115–S120
43. Bruix J, Sherman M (2011) Management of hepatocellular carcinoma: an update. Hepatology 53(3):1020–1022
44. Pawlik TM, Esnaola NF, Vauthey JN (2004) Surgical treatment of hepatocellular carcinoma: similar long-term results despite geographic variations. Liver Transpl 10(2 Suppl 1):S74–S80
45. Toyoda H, Kumada T, Kiriyama S, Sone Y, Tanikawa M, Hisanaga Y, Yamaguchi A, Isogai M, Kaneoka Y, Washizu J (2005) Comparison of the usefulness of three staging systems for hepatocellular carcinoma (CLIP, BCLC, and JIS) in Japan. Am J Gastroenterol 100(8):1764–1771
46. Lewis RB, Lattin GE Jr, Paal E (2010) Pancreatic endocrine tumors: radiologic-clinicopathologic correlation. Radiographics 30(6):1445–1464
47. Bielenberg DR, Zetter BR (2015) The contribution of angiogenesis to the process of metastasis. Cancer J 21(4):267–273
48. Migliozzi MT, Mucka P, Bielenberg DR (2014) Lymphangiogenesis and metastasis-a closer look at the neuropilin/semaphorin3 axis. Microvasc Res 96:68–76
49. Gomes FG, Nedel F, Alves AM, Nör JE, Tarquinio SBC (2013) Tumor angiogenesis and lymphangiogenesis: tumor/endothelial crosstalk and cellular/environmental signaling mechanisms. Life Sci 92:101–107
50. Ji RC (2006) Lymphatic endothelial cells, tumor lymphangiogenesis and metastasis: new insights into intratumoral and peritumoral lymphatics. Cancer Metastasis Rev 25:677–694
51. Nathanson SD (2003) Insights into the mechanisms of lymph node metastasis. Cancer 98(2):413–423

1

52. Shields JD, Emmett MS, Dunn DB, Joory KD, Sage LM, Rigby H, Mortimer PS, Orlando A, Levick JR, Bates DO (2007) Chemokine-mediated migration of melanoma cells towards lymphatics–a mechanism contributing to metastasis. Oncogene 26(21):2997–3005

53. Morton DL, Wen DR, Wong JH et al (1992) Technical details of intraoperative lymphatic mapping for early stage melanoma. Arch Surg 127:392–399

54. Krag DN, Meijer SJ, Weaver DL et al (1995) Minimal-access surgery for staging of malignant melanoma. Arch Surg 130:654–658

55. Fidler IJ (1970) Metastasis: quantitative analysis of distribution and fate of tumor embolilabeled with 125 I-5-iodo-2′-deoxyuridine. J Natl Cancer Inst 45(4): 773–782

56. Luzzi KJ et al (1998) Multistep nature of metastatic inefficiency: dormancy of solitary cells after successful extravasation and limited survival of early micrometastases. Am J Pathol 153:865–873

57. Guillerey C, Smyth MJ (2016) NK cells and cancer immunoediting. Curr Top Microbiol Immunol 395: 115–145

58. Chambers AF, Groom AC, MacDonald IC (2002) Dissemination and growth of cancer cells in metastatic sites. Nat Rev Cancer 2(8):563–572

59. Hedley BD, Chambers AF (2009) Tumor dormancy and metastasis. Adv Cancer Res 102:67–101

60. Weinberg RA (2006) The biology of cancer. Garland Science, New York

61. Paget S (1889) The distribution of secondary growths in cancer of the breast. Lancet 1:99–101

62. Ewing J (1928) Neoplastic diseases. A treatise on tumors. W.B. Saunders, Philadelphia, pp 77–89

63. Hart IR (1982) 'Seed and soil' revisited: mechanisms of sitespecific metastasis. Cancer Metastasis Rev 1:5–16

64. Zetter BR (1990) The cellular basis of site-specific tumor metastasis. N Engl J Med 322:605–612

65. Fidler IJ (2001) Seed and soil revisited: contribution of the organ microenvironment to cancer metastasis. Surg Oncol Clin N Am 10:257–269

66. Langley RR, Fidler IJ (2011) The seed and soil hypothesis revisited--the role of tumor-stroma interactions in metastasis to different organs. Int J Cancer 128(11): 2527–2535

67. Nguyen DX, Bos PD, Massagué J (2009) Metastasis: from dissemination to organ-specific colonization. Nat Rev Cancer 9(4):274–284

68. Ambrosetti MC, Zamboni GA, Mucelli RP (2016) Distribution of liver metastases based on the site of primary pancreatic carcinoma. Eur Radiol 26(2):306–310

69. Nieto J, Grossbard ML, Kozuch P (2008) Metastatic pancreatic cancer 2008: is the glass less empty? Oncologist 13(5):562–576

70. Okua K (1997) Hepatocellular carcinoma: clinicopathological aspects. J Gastroenterol Hepatol 12(9–10): S314–S318

71. Amit M, Na'ara S, Gil Z (2016) Mechanisms of cancer dissemination along nerves. Nat Rev Cancer 16(6):399–408

72. Batsakis JG (1985) Nerves and neurotropic carcinomas. Ann Otol Rhinol Laryngol 94(4 pt 1):426–427

73. Cruveilheir J (1835) Maladies Des Nerfs Anatomie Pathologique Du Corps Humain. JB Bailliere, Paris

74. Fagan JJ, Collins B, Barnes L et al (1998) Perineural invasion in squamous cell carcinoma of the head and neck. Arch Otolaryngol Head Neck Surg 124:637–640

75. Bockman DE, Buchler M, Beger HG (1994) Interaction of pancreatic ductal carcinoma with nerves leads to nerve damage. Gastroenterology 107:219–230

76. Nagakawa T, Kayahara M, Ohta T et al (1991) Patterns of neural and plexus invasion of human pancreatic cancer and experimental cancer. Int J Pancreatol 10:113–119

77. Larson DL, Rodin AE, Roberts DK, O'Steen WK, Rapperport AS, Lewis SR (1966) Perineural lymphatics: myth or fact. Am J Surg 112(4):488–492

78. Akert K, Sandri C, Weibel ER, Peper K, Moor H (1976) The fine structure of the perineural endothelium. Cell Tissue Res 165(3):281–295

79. Hassan MO, Maksem J (1980) The prostatic perineural space and its relation to tumor spread: an ultrastructural study. Am J Surg Pathol 4:143–148

80. Rodin AE, Larson DL, Roberts DK (1967) Nature of the perineural space invaded by prostatic carcinoma. Cancer 20:1772–1779

81. Bakst RL, Wong RJ (2016) Mechanisms of Perineural Invasion. J Neurol Surg B 77:96–106

82. Liebig C, Ayala G, Wilks JA, Berger DH, Albo D (2009) Perineural invasion in cancer: a review of the literature. Cancer 115(15):3379–3391

83. Marchesi F, Piemonti L, Mantovani A, Allavena P (2010) Molecular mechanisms of perineural invasion, a forgotten pathway of dissemination and metastasis. Cytokine Growth Factor Rev 21(1):77–82

84. Amit M et al (2015) International collaborative validation of intraneural invasion as a prognostic marker in adenoid cystic carcinoma of the head and neck. Head Neck 37:1038–1045

85. Ozaki H, Hiraoka T, Mizumoto R et al (1999) The prognostic significance of lymph node metastasis and intrapancreatic perineural invasion in pancreatic cancer after curative resection. Surg Today 29:16–22

Radiological Signs of Tumor Dissemination

Daniele Regge, Giovanni Cappello, and Giulia Zamboni

© Springer International Publishing AG 2018
D. Regge, G. Zamboni (eds.), *Hepatobiliary and Pancreatic Cancer*,
Cancer Dissemination Pathways, https://doi.org/10.1007/978-3-319-50296-0_2

2

2.1 Introduction

Assessment of tumor spread by imaging is important for treatment planning and to predict patient prognosis. Most significantly, imaging findings allow tailoring of surgical resection to the individual patient. For example, when imaging shows hepatocellular carcinoma (HCC) confined to one or few liver segments, patients can undergo parenchyma-sparing surgery allowing them to retain sufficient liver functionality even when chronic disease is present. Conversely, by identifying signs of locally advanced disease or distant metastases, oncologists may have but the option of neoadjuvant therapy or of palliative treatment, sparing unnecessary surgery to the patient.

Ultrasound (US) has a minor role in the assessment of tumor spread, due to its narrow field of view. However, it remains the primary imaging test for the surveillance of patients at risk for developing tumors in the abdominal parenchymas, e.g., the liver for HCC or metastases [1]. *Computed tomography* (CT) and *magnetic resonance imaging* (MRI) are the main imaging techniques for tumor diagnosis and staging; the latter may depict tumor functional characteristics and relate them to tumor aggressiveness. CT is usually the primary imaging test for staging of hepatobiliary and pancreatic neoplasia as it allows wide body coverage and has a high spatial resolution. Conversely, MRI's excellent contrast resolution allows better characterization of liver and pancreatic tumors, depiction of satellite nodules, and accurate assessment of tumor spread along the bile ducts.

Staging systems classify tumors according to the extent of their dissemination. Cancer staging allows clinicians to select the best treatment for each patient and provide prognostic information. The most commonly used staging system is the TNM devised by the French surgeon Pierre Denoix in 1943, developed and maintained by the Union for International Cancer Control (UICC) [2]. In the TNM system, T describes the primary tumor and the extent to which it invades the surrounding tissues, N describes the regional lymph node involvement, and M describes the presence or otherwise of distant metastases. TNM was initially adopted both by surgeons (cTNM) and pathologists (pTNM) to stage common solid tumors. With the advent of cross-sectional techniques, imaging criteria have been included in staging systems. TNM and other staging systems developed for hepatobiliary and pancreatic tumors will be discussed in the specific chapters.

2.2 Local Spread

As aforementioned, local spread is defined as the diffusion of a tumor within an organ or to adjacent structures by contiguity. The molecular mechanisms of local tumor spread are now largely known and so is their pathological appearance. In comparison to macroscopic pathological tumor sections, radiological images have a low resolution. Even though imaging signs of local dissemination are gross, they are usually sufficient to assess tumor extent in most cases. In this section, radiological signs of expansive and infiltrative local tumor spread and correlation with pathological features will be described.

2.2.1 Expansive Growth

Many liver and pancreatic tumors have an expansive growth pattern and may be surrounded by a capsule, usually composed of predominantly fibrous tissue containing thin vascular channels [3] or by a pseudocapsule formed by mixed fibrous tissue due to the compression of the tumor on the surrounding parenchyma or by hepatic sinusoids [4, 5]. At CT and MRI, the capsule typically shows a low-attenuating/hypointense rim on the arterial phase and is high-attenuating/hyperintense on the portal venous and on delayed phase images due to the retention of the slow-flowing contrast agent within the peritumoral microvessels [5, 6] (◘ Fig. 2.1). In progressed HCC, the presence of a capsule favors minimally invasive approaches to treatment and has a favorable prognosis in comparison to HCCs of similar grade but without or with a disrupted capsule [7–9]. Cystic tumors are frequently encapsulated and have smooth margins, and capsule imaging features may correlate with risk of malignancy. For example, thick-walled mucinous cystic tumors of the pancreas have a higher risk of malignancy than thin-walled lesions [10] (◘ Fig. 2.2).

Tumors without a capsule may also exhibit an expansive behavior. iCC that present with abundant fibrous stroma in the lesion center and a

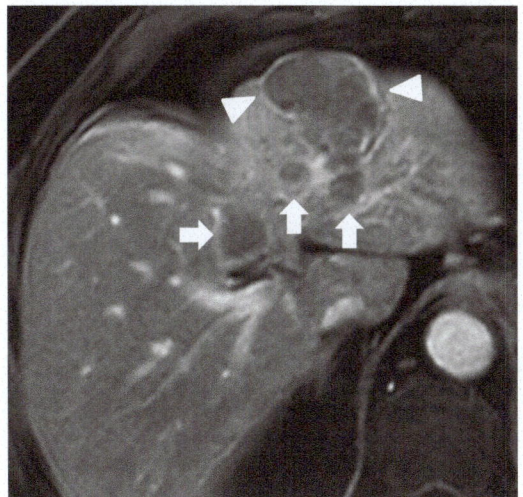

▣ Fig. 2.1 MR T1-weighted image during i.v. administration of gadolinium chelates. The image shows a case of advanced HCC. Dominant lesion in segment 3 is surrounded by a thin hyperintense capsule (*arrowheads*) which is disrupted posteriorly. Three satellite nodules can be appreciated not far from the primary lesion, in segments 3 and 4 (*white arrows*)

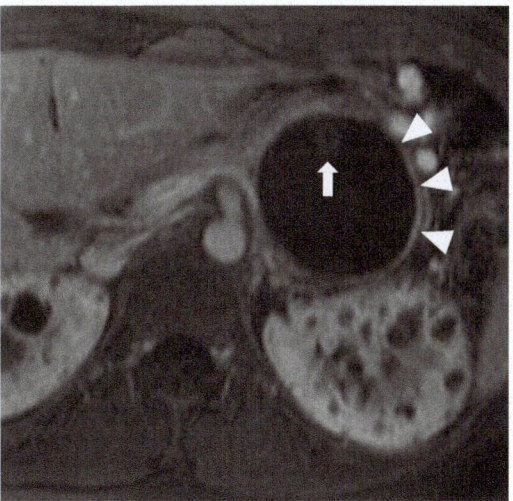

▣ Fig. 2.2 MR T1-weighted image during i.v. administration of gadolinium chelates. The image shows a case of mucinous cystic neoplasm of the tail of the pancreas. The presence of a thin enhancing capsule surrounding the lesion is a sign of benignity (*arrowheads*). A parietal nodule can be appreciated on the anterior border of the cystic lesion (*white arrow*)

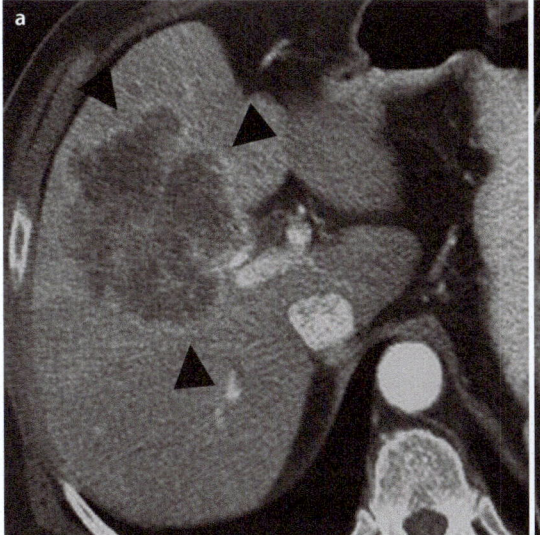

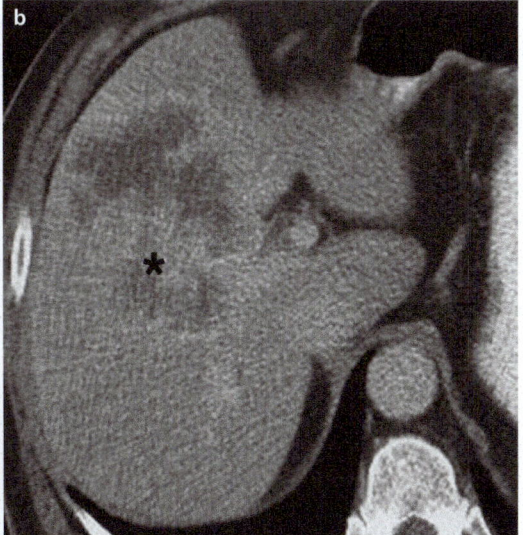

▣ Fig. 2.3 CT scan shows a large tumor involving segments 4 and 5. a Late arterial phase shows an inhomogeneous lesion with a gross irregular hyperdense pseudocapsule (*arrowheads*). b Delayed phase. The lesion retains contrast in its central part (*asterisk*). Diagnosis of iCC

greater density of viable cells at the tumor periphery usually show well-demarcated margins, early peripheral enhancement, and progression of enhancement toward the lesion center in the delayed phase [11] (▣ Fig. 2.3).

Patient prognosis worsens when microvascular invasion is present. According to Lin et al. [12], MVI is a more accurate predictor of tumor recurrence than the Milan criteria following surgical resection for HCC. Disruption

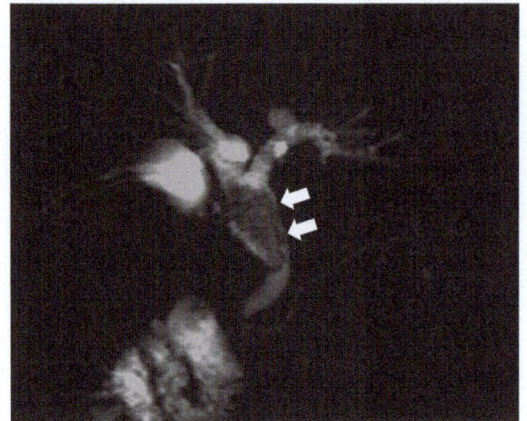

Fig. 2.4 MR cholangiopancreatography shows a large filling defect within the main bile duct with irregular margins (*white arrows*). Diagnosis of intraductal papillary bile duct neoplasm

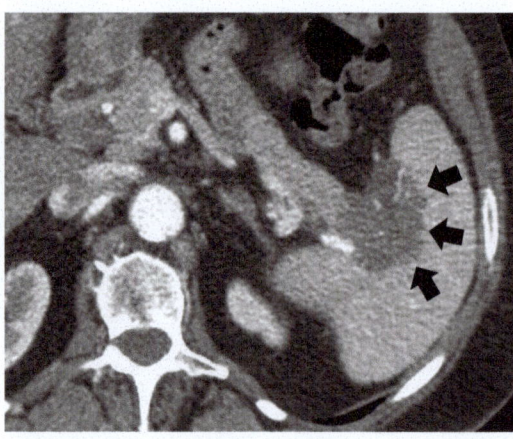

Fig. 2.5 Portal phase CT scan: NET of the pancreatic tail infiltrating the splenic parenchyma (*black arrows*)

of the capsule is an early sign of MVI and can be visible at imaging, as can invasion of surrounding tissues (Fig. 2.1). Signs of extracapsular extension of liver tumors such as corona enhancement, satellite nodules, and liver capsule retraction will be discussed in the specific chapters.

Bile duct cancer may occasionally present as an intraluminal polypoid mass and exhibit a benign behavior. Intraluminal expansive growth can be easily detected on conventional imaging, which usually shows a well-defined, round, or oval shape mass, with a sessile or cauliflower-like appearance extending within the bile duct lumen [13] (Fig. 2.4).

2.2.2 Infiltrative Growth

Tumors with an aggressive behavior invade and destroy the tissue within the organ of origin and spread beyond, infiltrating adjacent organs and structures by contiguity. In case of infiltrative growth, the role of imaging is to assess the extent of invasion and examine the relationship of the primary tumor with adjacent structures. At CT and MRI, the newly formed tissue does not present smooth margins, but conversely it is characterized by irregular digitations that expand within and beyond the affected organ (Fig. 2.5). When desmoplastic reaction and marked fibrosis are prevalent

and vital cells are a minority, as is the case of infiltrating pancreatic ductal adenocarcinoma (PDAC), tumor typically presents as a hypoattenuating/hypointense mass, with the best contrast between tumor and pancreatic parenchyma provided by CT or MRI during the pancreatic phase [14–16] (Fig. 2.6). Moreover, when cancer cells blend with the surrounding parenchima, tumors may present as inhomogeneous ill-defined masses. For example, when infiltrative subtype HCC cells intermingle with the regenerative substrate, the lesion is poorly vascularized and difficult to identify unless portal venous invasion is present [1] (Fig. 2.7).

Small infiltrating tumors may be difficult to identify by imaging, and indirect signs of the newly formed tissue must therefore be carefully sought. Small PDAC is frequently accompanied by indirect signs, such as the dilatation of the main pancreatic duct or the common bile duct, parenchymal atrophy, deformity of the pancreatic contours, and the loss of parenchymal lobulations [16, 17] (Fig. 2.8).

Extrahepatic cholangiocarcinoma (eCC) originates from the bile duct or gallbladder epithelium and has different growth patterns [13, 18]. The infiltrative pattern accounts for approximately two-thirds of bile duct cholangiocarcinomas [13]. In the latter case, tumor grows along the bile duct causing stenosis and/or a complete obliteration of its lumen [19]. When infiltrative behavior is present, CT and MRI show increased duct wall thick-

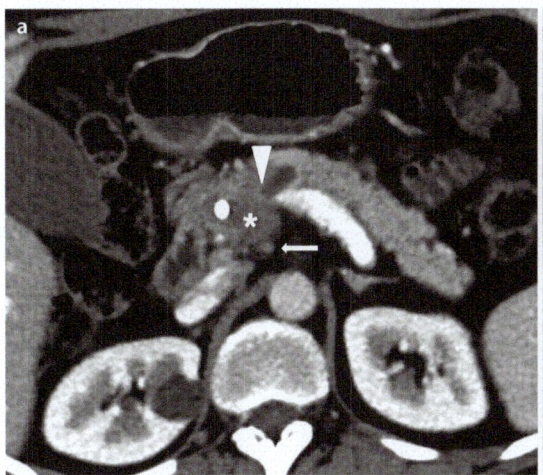 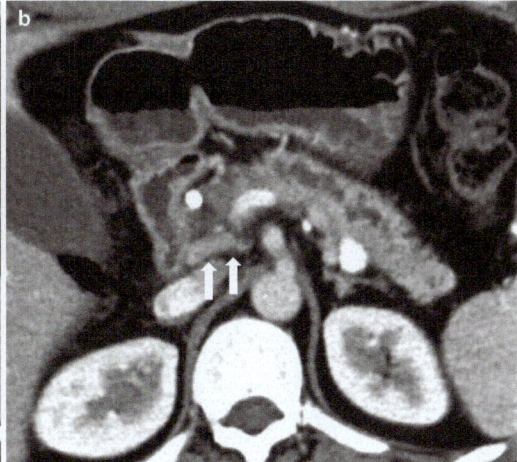

Fig. 2.6 Pancreatic phase CT scan: PDAC of the head. **a** The image shows a markedly hypoattenuating mass of the head of the pancreas (*asterisk*) infiltrating the main pancreatic duct and the portal vein (*white arrowhead*). The nodular extension of tumor into the medial-posterior fat area of the pancreatic head (*small arrow*) is a sign of perineural invasion. **b** The image shows an elongated enhancing lymph node of the fatty space located posteriorly to the pancreatic head (*white arrows*)

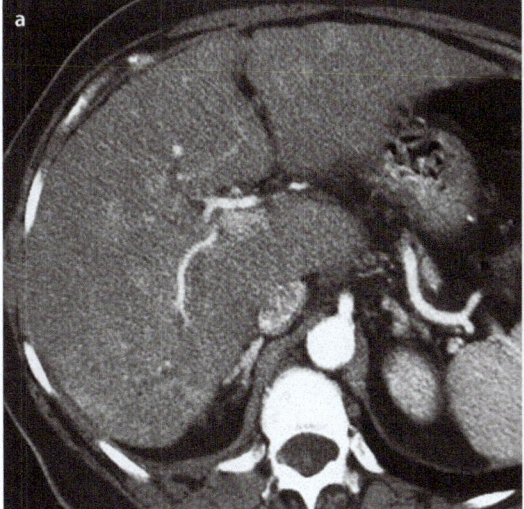 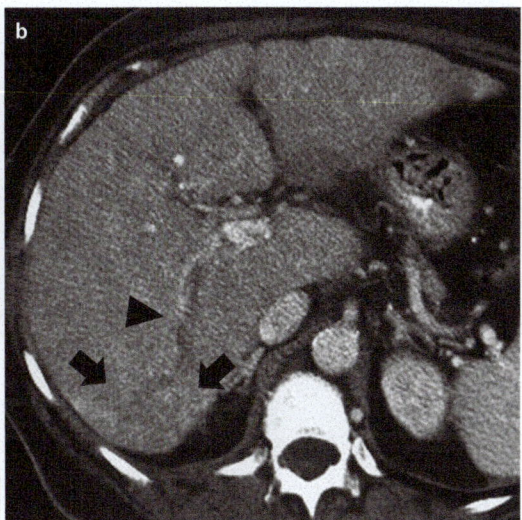

Fig. 2.7 Female, asymptomatic, αFP = 500. **a** Arterial phase. No focal lesions are visible on the CT scan. Of note, the right liver is slightly inhomogeneous. **b** Portal phase. CT scan shows a slightly hypodense region with ill-defined margins in segments 6 and 7 (*black arrows*). A large filling defect can be observed obstructing the right branch of the portal vein (*arrowhead point*). Diagnosis: infiltrating type HCC with intraluminal thrombosis

ness (duct wall >2 mm), arterial and/or portal phase wall enhancement (enhancing ring), and stenosis with dilatation of the biliary tree proximal to the lesion [20] (Fig. 2.9). Infiltrative type eCC may grow beyond the bile duct wall and invade the periductal fat tissue, the liver parenchyma, or the vessels of the hepatic pedicle [20]. Gallbladder carcinoma also has an infiltrative behavior in approximately two-thirds of cases [13]. As mentioned in the previous chapter, the absence of the submucosal layer and the irregular presence of the muscular layer favor invasion of the adjacent structures,

2

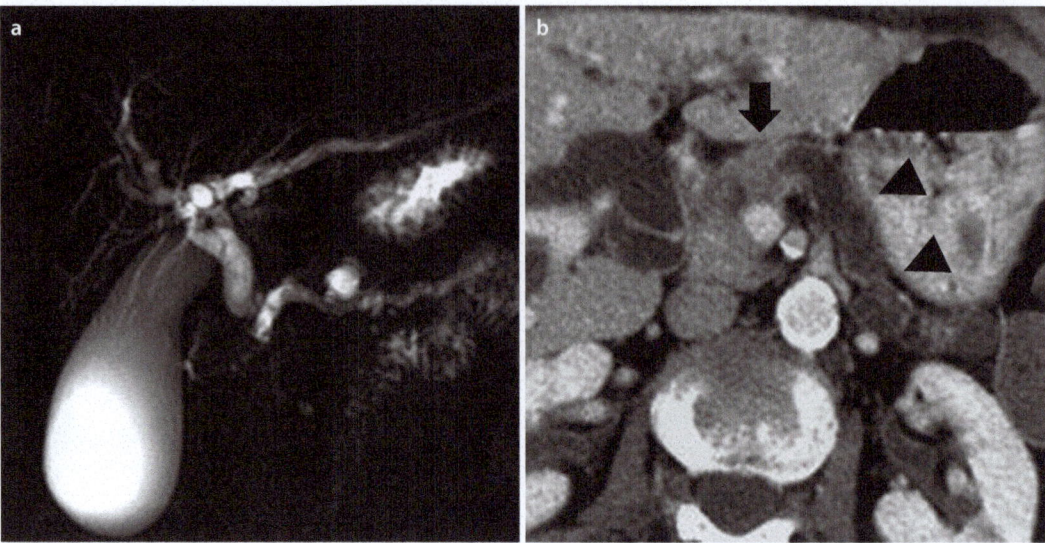

☐ **Fig. 2.8** Indirect signs of PDAC. **a** MRCP shows sharp narrowing of the distal main bile duct and of the pancreatic duct and dilatation of duct segments located proximally to the stenosis. **b** Pancreatic phase CT scan shows dilatation of the pancreatic duct and parenchymal atrophy (*black arrowheads*). The pancreatic parenchyma is slightly thickened at the level of the head with loss of lobulation (*black arrow*)

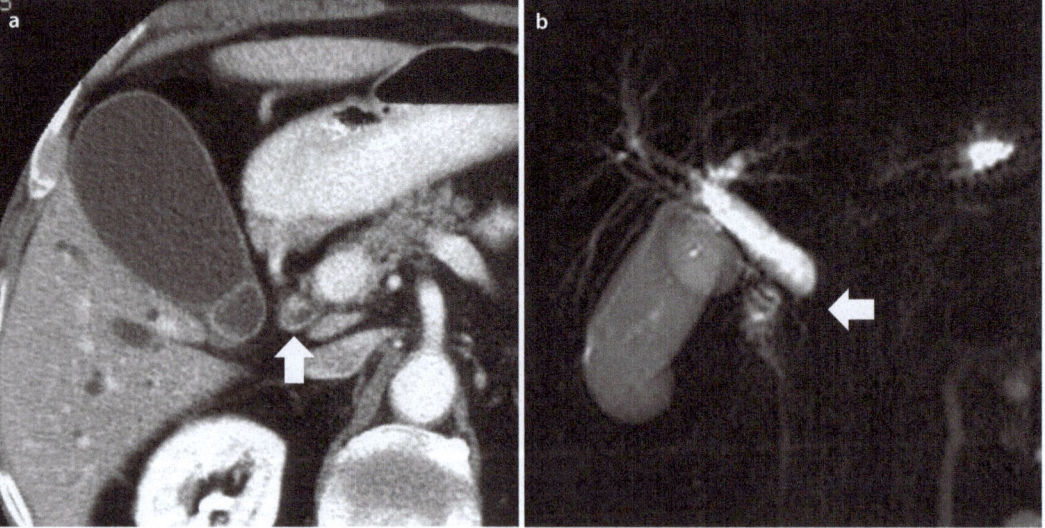

☐ **Fig. 2.9   a** Portal phase CT scan. White arrow points to the main bile duct that has thickened walls with ring like enhancement. **b** MRCP shows sharp narrowing of the distal main bile duct (*white arrow*) and dilatation of the proximal segments of the main bile duct, of the intrahepatic bile ducts and of the gallbladder. Diagnosis of eCC

frequently present at the time of diagnosis [13, 21–23]. At CT, gallbladder carcinoma typically presents as a hypo- to isoattenuating mass, which may contain low-attenuation areas of necrosis as well as enhancing foci of viable tumor (☐ Figs. 2.10 and 2.11). At MRI, the tumor is characterized by hypointensity on the T1-weighted images and hyperintensity on the T2-weighted images, with ill-defined early enhancement on gadolinium-enhanced images. MRCP may be useful for the evaluation of the extent of biliary duct invasion [19, 23] (□ Fig. 2.11). Both CT and MR imaging also provide information on the eventual encroachment of tumor tissue in the liver or in other surrounding structures (□ Figs. 2.10 and 2.11).

2.3 Vascular Invasion

The migration of tumor cells into the vessel lumen (i.e., intravasation [24]) is a characteristic of advanced tumors [3, 5]. Intravasation provides a route for tumor dissemination and aggravates patient prognosis [3, 5]. HCC [5] and occasionally pancreatic neuroendocrine tumors (PNETs) may invade the portal vein and develop intraluminal thrombosis (□ Fig. 2.7). Conversely, other histotypes of hepatobiliary and pancreatic cancers infiltrate the wall of arteries and veins from the outside causing luminal narrowing. Vascular infiltration affects staging and treatment strategy. PDAC, for example, is defined as locally advanced, therefore not amenable to surgery, if encasement of more than 180° of the circumference of the superior mesenteric artery or of celiac arteries by tumor is present at cross-sectional imaging [17, 25]. Vascular invasion frequently represents the line of demarcation between radical surgery and palliative treatment.

When small vessels are involved, vascular invasion can be detected only at microscopy. Conversely, imaging has a fundamental role in the assessment of macroscopic vascular invasion, i.e., the extension of tumor tissue inside a vessel (□ Fig. 2.7) and of vascular encasement

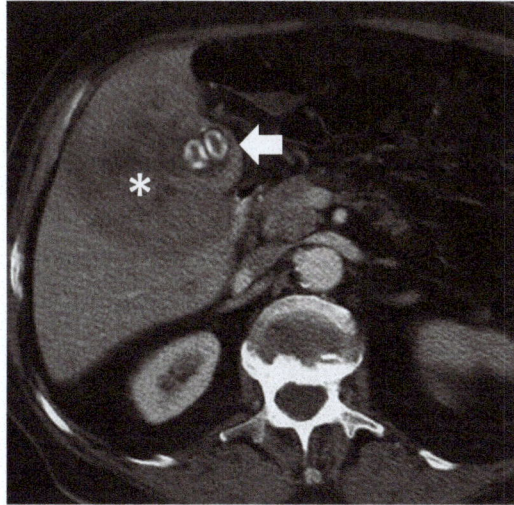

□ **Fig. 2.10** Portal phase CT scan. Large inhomogeneous hypoattenuating mass arising from the gallbladder and extensively infiltrating the liver parenchyma (*asterisk*). The arrow points to two large gallbladder stones. Diagnosis of gallbladder carcinoma

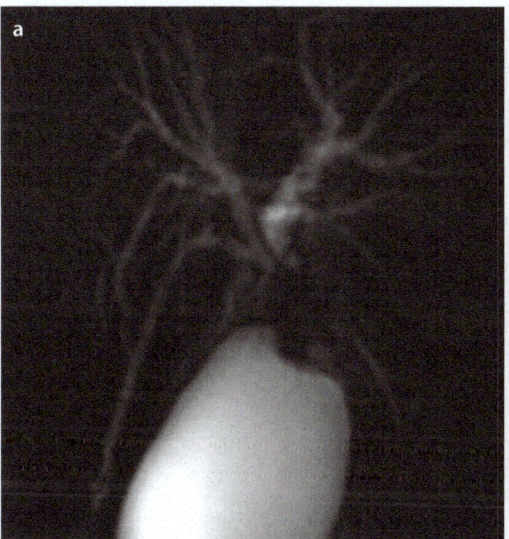
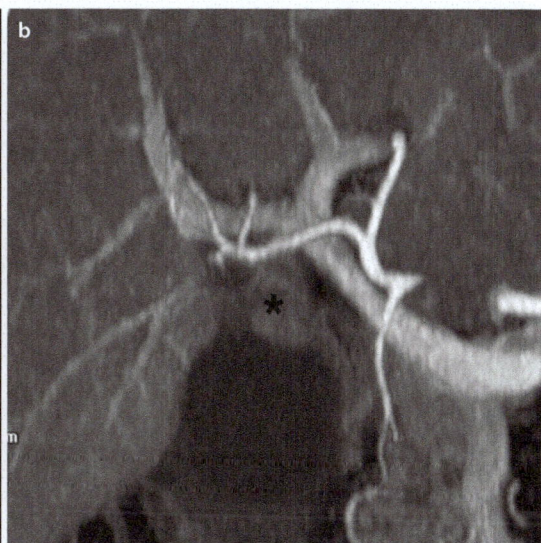

□ **Fig. 2.11** **a** MRCP shows a filling defect at the level of the gallbladder neck, a signal void corresponding to the proximal main bile duct and dilatation of the intrahepatic bile ducts. **b** Coronal CT maximum intensity projection shows a solid lesion of the gallbladder neck (*asterisk*). Diagnosis of gallbladder carcinoma

2

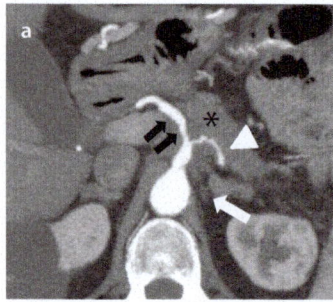
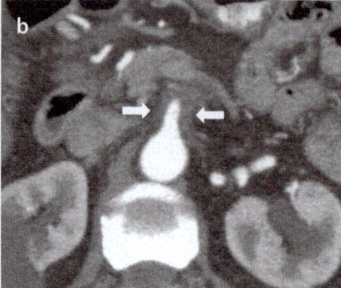
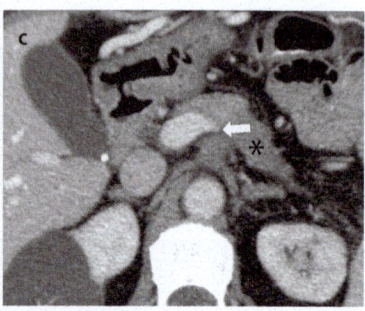

◘ **Fig. 2.12**   **a** Arterial phase CT scan: PDAC of the body-tail. The image shows a hypoattenuating mass of the body-tail of the pancreas (*asterisk*) encasing the splenic artery (*white arrowhead*) and the common hepatic artery (*black arrows*). Posteriorly the tumor infiltrates the peripancreatic fat and extends to the left celiac ganglia (*white arrow*). **b** Same patient, arterial phase CT scan. Note the encasement of the superior mesenteric artery and the infiltration of the celiac plexus by the tumor (*white arrows*). **c** Same patient, portal phase CT scan. The *white arrow* shows the "teardrop appearance" of the portal vein due to compression by the tumor (*asterisk*)

(◘ Fig. 2.12). While intraluminal thrombosis is easy to identify at imaging, the true challenge remains to distinguish between a true tumor thrombus and a bland thrombus that has a different therapeutic approach and prognosis [26, 27]. The presence of a gross direct extension of a parenchymal tumor in an adjacent vessel [4], of neovascularity inside the thrombus, usually with the same characteristics of the main tumor, and punctate hyperenhancing "threads and streaks" within the vessel are characteristic imaging features of tumor thrombus [4, 27] (◘ Fig. 2.7). In equivocal cases, MR DWI sequences may provide assistance in the differentiation of the two entities, a restricted signal being observed in case of neoplastic thrombus [26]. Tublin et al. report a lumen dilation threshold of 23 mm to identify a tumor thrombus [27]. However, it should be noted that vascular expansion may be present also in acute bland thrombosis [4] in patients with portal hypertension [26].

The presence of a fat plane between the tumor and a vessel (◘ Fig. 2.13) excludes the presence of vascular invasion [17]. In case a direct contact between the newly formed tissue and a vessel is appreciated at cross-sectional imaging, the role of the radiologist is to describe in detail the relationship between the tumor and the adjacent major vascular structures [17]. In fact, the extent of the tumor tissue around a vessel correlates with the probability of vessel invasion [28]. The term "abutment" characterize a tumor-vessel connection in which tumor involves <50% (<180°) of the vessel circumference (◘ Fig. 2.14). Conversely, "encasement" is defined when a vessel is surrounded by

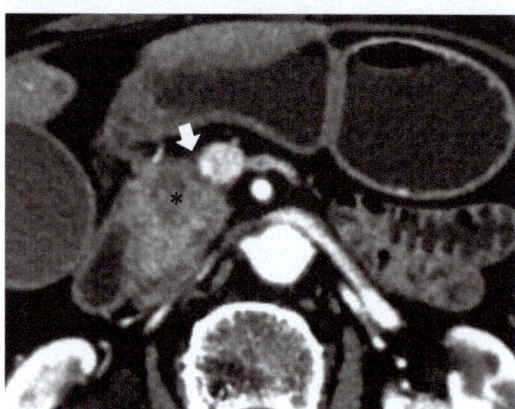

◘ **Fig. 2.13**   Pancreatic phase CT image shows a moderately hypoattenuating lesion of the pancreatic head (*asterisk*). The thin hypodense line between the lesion and the superior mesenteric vein (*arrow*) is a fatty plane that excludes the presence of vascular invasion

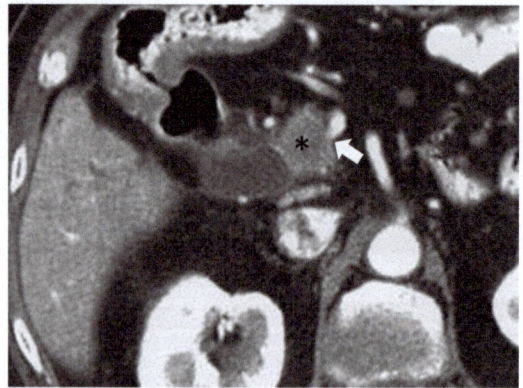

◘ **Fig. 2.14**   Pancreatic phase CT scan. The image shows an hypoattenuating mass of the head of the pancreas (*asterisk*). The tumor-vessel contact (*white arrow*) is <50% of the circumference of the vessel ("abutment")

more than 50% (>180°) by tumor tissue [28] (◘ Fig. 2.12). A CT grading system has been proposed to measure vascular involvement in PDAC [29] (◘ Table 2.1) where a 100% probability of vessel invasion has been observed in case of encasement >270° [17].

In pancreatic head tumor, a particular sign that is occasionally detected with imaging is the "teardrop" appearance of the superior mesenteric or portal vein [17, 28] (◘ Fig. 2.12c), a sign that is strongly related to tumor-vessel infiltration and considered a reliable indicator of unresectability, even if other signs are absent. In fact, in their retrospective study, Hough et al. found the SMV "teardrop" appearance as the only sign of nonresectability in 13 of 17 patients [30].

◘ **Table 2.1** CT grading system for the assessment of vascular involvement in PDAC [29]

Grade	Tumor-vessel contact	Chance of vessel invasion
0	Absent	0%
1	<90°	0–3%
2	90–180°	~40% (29–57%)
3	>180°	~80%

2.4 Lymphatic Involvement

In hepatobiliary and pancreatic cancer, lymphatic involvement is an important determinant of patient survival and may affect treatment planning [31]. It is therefore mandatory to perform accurate evaluation of nodal status.

At cross-sectional imaging, normal lymph nodes present smooth and well-defined margins, oval or cigar-like shape, a central fatty hilum, and have uniform and homogeneous density or signal intensity [32]. According to most imaging criteria, lymph nodes are considered metastatic when their short axis is >1 cm [33]. For hepatobiliary and pancreatic tumors, however, size criteria alone are unreliable in the assessment of the lymph node status. Noji et al. [34] evaluated regional lymph node metastases with CT in 146 patients with biliary cancer that underwent lymphadenectomy. They showed that only 28% of hepatoduodenal ligament lymph nodes with a short axis >1 cm were infiltrated by cancer [34] (◘ Fig. 2.15b). Indeed, lymph node hyperplasia, a common finding in patients with liver chronic disease or infection, may also cause hilar lymph node enlargement [34]. Dodd et al. examined 507 patients with end-stage cirrhosis for enlarged lymph nodes [35]. They found that 50% of subjects (253/507) had lymph nodes with a short axis >1 cm, including 36 of the 58 patients with cancer in the series. Of the latter, only two had

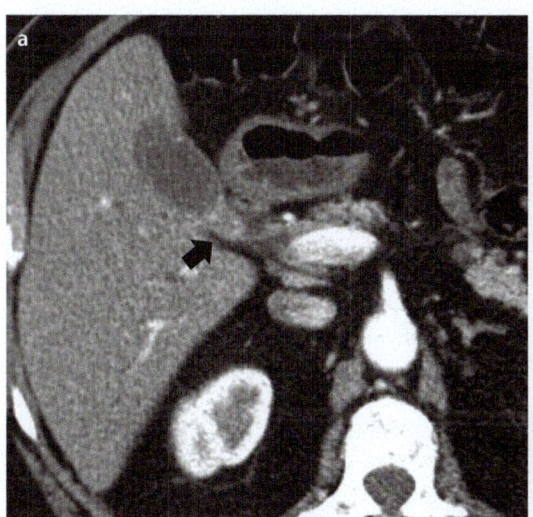
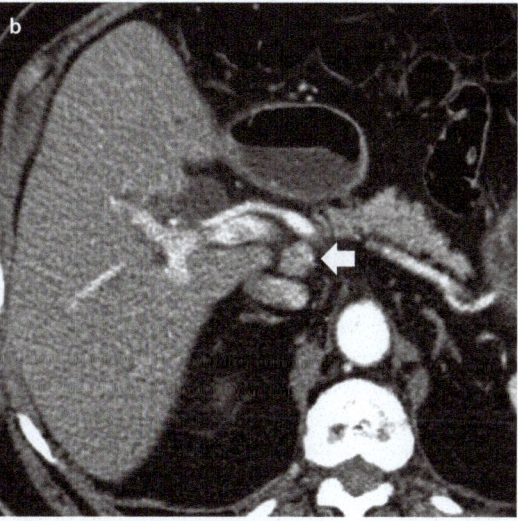

◘ **Fig. 2.15** Arterial phase CT shows **a** a solid round lesion of the gallbladder neck (*black arrow*) and **b** a 15 mm enhancing lymph node of the hepatic pedicle, posterior to the common hepatic artery. Diagnosis of gallbladder carcinoma with lymph node metastases

2

metastatic lymph nodes, while the remaining revealed a benign reactive process at histology [35].

Heterogeneous enhancement of lymph node internal structure is a more specific sign of tumor involvement. In their series Noji et al. found that 64% of lymph nodes with a heterogeneous pattern were metastatic [34]. Ringlike enhancement appears to be even more specific for metastatic involvement than the heterogeneous pattern but is rarely encountered [36].

Conversely, for PDAC, nodules of the fat area surrounding the pancreas should raise suspicion of lymph node neoplastic involvement (● Fig. 2.6b). Mochizuki et al. [37] correlated CT findings with those of en bloc pathological specimens from resected pancreatic tumor. They detected 95 lymph nodes with a short axis <1 cm in the medial posterior area of the pancreas head in a total of 28 patients, of whom 14 (15%) with metastases [37]. Overall, detection and characterization of lymph node metastases by CT yield disappointing results.

At MRI, metastatic lymph nodes are hyperintense on T2-weighted fat-suppressed images and show inhomogeneous enhancement on T1-weighted post-contrast images [38, 39]. Diffusion-weighted imaging may help characterize abdominal lymph nodes. Lower ADC values were observed by Akudman et al. in malignant lymph nodes in comparison to those with benign histology [40].

Summarizing, today's imaging technology is insufficient to predict lymph node status in the context of hepatobiliary and pancreatic tumors. Further technical advances, such as improvement of spatial and temporal resolution of available imaging modalities or the implementation of new contrast agents, might in the future allow reliable detection and characterization of benign and malignant lymph nodes.

2.5 Perineural Invasion

Perineural invasion (PNI) is one of the most important prognostic factors in hepatobiliary and pancreatic tumors. Despite its importance, PNI is not included in most staging systems. PNI is present at histopathologic examination in up to 80–91% of resected iCC [41] and PDAC, respectively [42]. Unfortunately, direct invasion of the nerve sheath is not evaluable with conventional imaging and can only be confirmed by the pathologist. However, the presence of tumor along the

nervous pathways at imaging should be considered highly suspicious of PNI.

The liver and the biliary tree are innervated by autonomic nerve fibers that run along major hepatic arteries within the hepatoduodenal ligament (hepatic artery) and gastrohepatic ligament (left gastric artery) [43]. Neurovascular bundles originate from the celiac ganglia and reach the abovementioned ligaments via the celiac plexus. The pancreatic head and the uncinate process are surrounded by a rich network of nerves, called plexus pancreaticus capitalis (PC) 1 and 2, described for the first time by Yoshioka and Wakabayashi [44]. PC1 originates from the right coeliac ganglion and extends along the posterior border of the pancreatic head behind the portal vein to enter the medial aspect of the uncinated process [45]. PC2 runs caudally to PC1, originates from the superior mesenteric artery plexus, and extends along the inferior pancreaticoduodenal artery and jejunal trunk [37, 46]. The latter is the preferential dissemination pathway of pancreatic adenocarcinoma of the uncinate process [45]. Finally, the tail and body of the pancreas are innerved by the splenic plexus [47, 48].

Multidetector computer tomography (MDCT) is the preferred imaging technique to detect PNI due to its high spatial and contrast resolution. On MDCT, PNI appears as soft tissue with the same density of tumor tissue, extending from the primary lesion along the neural pathways [45]. This results in streaky or strand-like structures within the fat tissue or in irregular masses near or in continuity with the tumor (● Fig. 2.6a). In adenocarcinoma of the pancreatic head, PNI progressively invades and cancels the adipose planes lying posteriorly and medially to the uncinate process and infiltrate the celiac ganglions. Ultimately, tissue may surround one or more of the following vessels: superior mesenteric artery, pancreaticoduodenal artery, superior mesenteric vein, celiac trunk, or splenic vein [49] (● Fig. 2.12a, b). In liver and bile duct tumors, PNI may show as a soft tissue mass or with a reticulate pattern within the hepatoduodenal or gastrohepatic ligaments and may surround the common hepatic artery or the left gastric artery.

In their study on the MDCT findings of extrapancreatic nerve plexus invasion by pancreas head carcinoma, Mochizuki et al. [37] describe four different CT patterns of peripancreatic tissue findings: fine reticular and linear, coarse reticular, mass and strand, and nodular. In fact, 92% of patients with mass and strand pattern and 63% of those with a coarse reticular pattern had PNI at pathology, suggesting that PNI should be reported when these patterns are detected on MDCT [37].

PNI is identified on MRI when either strand-like or mass-like signal intensity, like that of the original tumor, is detected along the neural pathways [49]. In pancreatic adenocarcinoma, PNI typically shows hypointense signal intensity on T1-weighted, iso- or moderate hyperintense signal on T2-weighted, hypointense signal on the arterial phase, and isointensity on the delayed phase images after Gd-DTPA contrast enhancement.

2.6 Distant Metastases

The presence of cancer cells in distant sites is a poor prognostic factor and contraindicates surgery in the large majority of patients with hepatobiliary and pancreatic malignancies [16]. Tumors with a more aggressive behavior usually present distant metastases at the time of diagnosis. Indeed, approximately 50% of PDAC are diagnosed late, when distant metastases are already present [14]. Conversely, more benign tumors such as mucinous cystic neoplasms have a far lower risk of metastatic dissemination [50].

Distant metastases are usually detected at cross-sectional imaging. CT is commonly adopted for staging purposes since it allows a high-resolution whole-body scan in a few seconds, while MRI is performed in specific clinical situations. For example, MRI with liver-specific contrast agent can be used to assess liver involvement since it has a higher sensitivity in the detection of small metastatic liver lesions in comparison to CT and PET [51]. Furthermore, MRI allows accurate characterization of indeterminate liver lesions [52]. Of note, secondary tumors usually present the same imaging characteristics of primary lesions. Hepatic metastases in patients with PDAC are hypovascular [14], while lung metastases from HCC present as soft tissue nodules which exhibit contrast enhancement in the arterial phase [53].

Positron emission tomography (PET) is not performed routinely in patients with hepatobiliary and pancreatic cancers [54]. However, PET/CT may support clinical decision-making in specific clinical conditions. In some borderline situations where surgeons are uncertain on whether to perform surgery or not, FDG-PET may support decision-making by detecting or excluding distant metastases in anatomical regions that are difficult to evaluate by CT and MRI, such as the peritoneal cavity or the bone [54]. Nuclear medicine is also useful in the context of pancreatic neuroendocrine tumours (PNET) that expresses somatostatin receptors. In particular, ^{68}Ga-labeled somatostatin analogues are helpful to localize primary tumor and detect sites of metastases [55–57].

References

1. Reynolds AR, Furlan A, Fetzer DT, Sasatomi E, Borhani AA, Heller MT, Tublin ME (2015) Infiltrative hepatocellular carcinoma: what radiologists need to know. Radiographics 35(2):371–386
2. Edge SB, Compton CC (2010) The American Joint Committee on Cancer: the 7th edition of the AJCC cancer staging manual and the future of the TNM. Ann Surg Oncol 17:1471–1474
3. Choi JY, Lee JM, Sirlin CB (2014) CT and MR imaging diagnosis and staging of hepatocellular carcinoma: part I. Development, growth, and spread: key pathologic and imaging aspects. Radiology 272(3):635–654
4. Choi JY, Lee JM, Sirlin CB (2014) CT and MR imaging diagnosis and staging of hepatocellular carcinoma: part II. Extracellular agents, hepatobiliary agents, and ancillary imaging features. Radiology 273(1):30–50
5. Cho ES, Choi JY (2015) MRI features of hepatocellular carcinoma related to biologic behavior. Korean J Radiol 16(3):449–464
6. Ünal E, İdilman İS, Akata D, Özmen MN, Karçaaltıncaba M (2016) Microvascular invasion in hepatocellular carcinoma. Diagn Interv Radiol 22(2):125–132
7. Ishigami K, Yoshimitsu K, Nishihara Y, Irie H, Asayama Y, Tajima T et al (2009) Hepatocellular carcinoma with a pseudocapsule on gadolinium-enhanced MR images: correlation with histopathologic findings. Radiology 250:435–443
8. Grazioli L, Olivetti L, Fugazzola C, Benetti A, Stanga C, Dettori E et al (1999) The pseudocapsule in hepatocellular carcinoma: correlation between dynamic MR imaging and pathology. Eur Radiol 9:62–67
9. Iguchi T, Aishima S, Sanefuji K, Fujita N, Sugimachi K, Gion T et al (2009) Both fibrous capsule formation and extracapsular penetration are powerful predictors of poor survival in human hepatocellular carcinoma: a histological assessment of 365 patients in Japan. Ann Surg Oncol 16:2539–2546
10. Procacci C, Carbognin G, Accordini S, Biasiutti C, Guarise A, Lombardo F, Ghirardi C, Graziani R, Pagnotta N, De Marco R (2001) CT features of malignant mucinous cystic tumors of the pancreas. Eur Radiol 11(9):1626–1630
11. Zhang Y, Uchida M, Abe T, Nishimura H, Hayabuchi N, Nakashima Y (1999) Intrahepatic peripheral

cholangiocarcinoma: comparison of dynamic CT and dynamic MRI. J Comput Assist Tomogr 23(5): 670–677

12. Lim KC, Chow PK, Allen JC et al (2011) Microvascular invasion is a better predictor of tumor recurrence and overall survival following surgical resection for hepatocellular carcinoma compared to the Milan criteria. Ann Surg 254:108–113

13. Levy AD, Murakata LA, Rohrmann CA Jr (2001) Gallbladder carcinoma: radiologic-pathologic correlation. Radiographics 21(2):295–314

14. Frampas E, David A, Regenet N, Touchefeu Y, Meyer J, Morla O (2016) Pancreatic carcinoma: key-points from diagnosis to treatment. Diagn Interv Imaging 97(12):1207–1223

15. Sahani DV, Shah ZK, Catalano OA, Boland GW, Brugge WR (2008) Radiology of pancreatic adenocarcinoma: current status of imaging. J Gastroenterol Hepatol 23(1):23–33

16. Pietryga JA, Morgan DE (2015) Imaging preoperatively for pancreatic adenocarcinoma. J Gastrointest Oncol 6(4):343–357

17. Schima W, Ba-Ssalamah A, Kölblinger C, Kulinna-Cosentini C, Puespoek A, Götzinger P (2007) Pancreatic adenocarcinoma. Eur Radiol 17(3):638–649

18. Nakanishi Y, Zen Y, Kawakami H, Kubota K, Itoh T, Hirano S, Tanaka E, Nakanuma Y, Kondo S (2008) Extrahepatic bile duct carcinoma with extensive intraepithelial spread: a clinicopathological study of 21 cases. Mod Pathol 21(7):807–816

19. Hennedige TP, Neo WT, Venkatesh SK (2014) Imaging of malignancies of the biliary tract-an update. Cancer Imaging 14:14

20. Engelbrecht MR, Katz SS, van Gulik TM, Laméris JS, van Delden OM (2015) Imaging of perihilar cholangiocarcinoma. AJR Am J Roentgenol 204(4):782–791

21. Yoshimitsu K, Honda H, Shinozaki K, Aibe H, Kuroiwa T, Irie H, Chijiiwa K, Asayama Y, Masuda K (2002) Helical CT of the local spread of carcinoma of the gallbladder: evaluation according to the TNM system in patients who underwent surgical resection. AJR Am J Roentgenol 179(2):423–428

22. Wistuba II, Gazdar AF (2004) Gallbladder cancer: lessons from a rare tumour. Nat Rev Cancer 4(9): 695–706

23. Hussain HM, Little MD, Wei S (2013) AIRP best cases in radiologic-pathologic correlation: gallbladder carcinoma with direct invasion of the liver. Radiographics 33(1):103–108

24. Leber MF, Efferth T (2009) Molecular principles of cancer invasion and metastasis (review). Int J Oncol 34(4):881–895

25. Vincent A, Herman J, Schulick R, Hruban RH, Goggins M (2011) Pancreatic cancer. Lancet 378(9791):607–620

26. Catalano OA, Choy G, Zhu A, Hahn PF, Sahani DV (2010) Differentiation of malignant thrombus from bland thrombus of the portal vein in patients with hepatocellular carcinoma: application of diffusion-weighted MR imaging. Radiology 254(1):154–162

27. Tublin ME, Dodd GD III, Baron RL (1997) Benign and malignant portal vein thrombosis: differentiation by CT characteristics. AJR Am J Roentgenol 168(3):719–723

28. Zakharova OP, Karmazanovsky GG, Egorov VI (2012) Pancreatic adenocarcinoma: outstanding problems. World J Gastrointest Surg 4(5):104–113

29. Lu DS, Reber HA, Krasny RM, Kadell BM, Sayre J (1997) Local staging of pancreatic cancer: criteria for unresectability of major vessels as revealed by pancreatic-phase, thin-section helical CT. AJR Am J Roentgenol 168(6):1439–1443

30. Hough TJ, Raptopoulos V, Siewert B, Matthews JB (1999) Teardrop superior mesenteric vein: CT sign for unresectable carcinoma of the pancreas. AJR Am J Roentgenol 173(6):1509–1512

31. Imai H, Doi R, Kanazawa H, Kamo N, Koizumi M, Masui T, Iwanaga Y, Kawaguchi Y, Takada Y, Isoda H, Uemoto S (2010) Preoperative assessment of para-aortic lymph node metastasis in patients with pancreatic cancer. Int J Clin Oncol 15(3):294–300

32. Torabi M, Aquino SL, Harisinghani MG (2004) Current concepts in lymph node imaging. J Nucl Med 45(9):1509–1518

33. Eisenhauer EA, Therasse P, Bogaerts J, Schwartz LH, Sargent D, Ford R, Dancey J, Arbuck S, Gwyther S, Mooney M, Rubinstein L, Shankar L, Dodd L, Kaplan R, Lacombe D, Verweij J (2009) New response evaluation criteria in solid tumours: revised RECIST guideline (version 1.1). Eur J Cancer 45(2):228–247

34. Noji T, Kondo S, Hirano S, Tanaka E, Suzuki O, Shichinohe T (2008) Computed tomography evaluation of regional lymph node metastases in patients with biliary cancer. Br J Surg 95(1):92–96

35. Dodd GD 3rd, Baron RL, Oliver JH 3rd, Federle MP, Baumgartel PB (1997) Enlarged abdominal lymph nodes in end-stage cirrhosis: CT-histopathologic correlation in 507 patients. Radiology 203(1):127–130

36. Ohtani T, Shirai Y, Tsukada K, Muto T, Hatakeyama K (1996) Spread of gallbladder carcinoma: CT evaluation with pathologic correlation. Abdom Imaging 21(3):195–201

37. Mochizuki K, Gabata T, Kozaka K, Hattori Y, Zen Y, Kitagawa H, Kayahara M, Ohta T, Matsui O (2010) MDCT findings of extrapancreatic nerve plexus invasion by pancreas head carcinoma: correlation with en bloc pathological specimens and diagnostic accuracy. Eur Radiol 20(7):1757–1767

38. Masselli G, Gualdi G (2008) Hilar cholangiocarcinoma: MRI/MRCP in staging and treatment planning. Abdom Imaging 33(4):444–451

39. Ringe KI, Wacker F (2015) Radiological diagnosis in cholangiocarcinoma: application of computed tomography, magnetic resonance imaging, and positron emission tomography. Best Pract Res Clin Gastroenterol 29(2):253–265

40. Akduman EI, Momtahen AJ, Balci NC, Mahajann N, Havlioglu N, Wolverson MK (2008) Comparison between malignant and benign abdominal lymph nodes on diffusion-weighted imaging. Acad Radiol 15(5):641–646

41. Raghavan K, Jeffrey RB, Patel BN, DiMaio MA, Willmann JK, Olcott EW (2015) MDCT diagnosis of perineural invasion involving the celiac plexus in intrahepatic cholangiocarcinoma: preliminary observations and clinical implications. AJR Am J Roentgenol 205(6):W578–W584

42. Kayahara M, Nagakawa T, Konishi I, Ueno K, Ohta T, Miyazaki I (1991) Clinicopathological study of pancreatic carcinoma with particular reference to the invasion of the extrapancreatic neural plexus. Int J Pancreatol 10(2):105–111

43. Ward EM, Rorie DK, Nauss LA, Bahn RC (1979) The celiac ganglia in man: normal anatomic variations. Anesth Analg 58(6):461–465

44. Yoshioka H, Wakabayashi T (1958) Therapeutic neurotomy on head of pancreas for relief of pain due to chronic pancreatitis; a new technical procedure and its results. AMA Arch Surg 76(4):546–554

45. Deshmukh SD, Willmann JK, Jeffrey RB (2010) Pathways of extrapancreatic perineural invasion by pancreatic adenocarcinoma: evaluation with 3D volume-rendered MDCT imaging. AJR Am J Roentgenol 194(3):668–674

46. Makino I, Kitagawa H, Ohta T et al (2008) Nerve plexus invasion in pancreatic cancer: spread patters on histopathologic and embryological analyses. Pancreas 37:358–365

47. Mitsunaga S, Hasebe T, Kinoshita T, Konishi M, Takahashi S, Gotohda N, Nakagohri T, Ochiai A (2007) Detail histologic analysis of nerve plexus invasion in invasive ductal carcinoma of the pancreas and its prognostic impact. Am J Surg Pathol 31(11):1636–1644

48. Yi SQ, Miwa K, Ohta T, Kayahara M, Kitagawa H, Tanaka A, Shimokawa T, Akita K, Tanaka S (2003) Innervation of the pancreas from the perspective of perineural invasion of pancreatic cancer. Pancreas 27(3):225–229

49. Zuo HD, Tang W, Zhang XM, Zhao QH, Xiao B (2012) CT and MR imaging patterns for pancreatic carcinoma invading the extrapancreatic neural plexus (part II): imaging of pancreatic carcinoma nerve invasion. World J Radiol 4(1):13–20

50. Crippa S, Salvia R, Warshaw AL, Domínguez I, Bassi C, Falconi M, Thayer SP, Zamboni G, Lauwers GY, Mino-Kenudson M, Capelli P, Pederzoli P, Castillo CF (2008) Mucinous cystic neoplasm of the pancreas is not an aggressive entity: lessons from 163 resected patients. Ann Surg 247(4):571–579

51. Motosugi U, Ichikawa T, Morisaka H et al (2011) Detection of pancreatic carcinoma and liver metastases with gadoxetic acid-enhanced MR imaging: comparison with contrast-enhanced multi-detector row CT. Radiology 260:446–453

52. Koelblinger C, Ba-Ssalamah A, Goetzinger P et al (2011) Gadobenate dimeglumine-enhanced 3.0-T MR imaging versus multiphasic 64-detector row CT: prospective evaluation in patients suspected of having pancreatic cancer. Radiology 259:757–766

53. Sneag DB, Krajewski K, Giardino A, O'Regan KN, Shinagare AB, Jagannathan JP, Ramaiya N (2011) Extrahepatic spread of hepatocellular carcinoma: spectrum of imaging findings. AJR Am J Roentgenol 197(4):W658–W664

54. Lan BY, Kwee SA, Wong LL (2012) Positron emission tomography in hepatobiliary and pancreatic malignancies: a review. Am J Surg 204(2):232–241

55. Bozkurt MF, Virgolini I, Balogova S, Beheshti M, Rubello D, Decristoforo C, Ambrosini V, Kjaer A, Delgado-Bolton R, Kunikowska J, Oyen WJG, Chiti A, Giammarile F, Fanti S (2017) Guideline for PET/CT imaging of neuroendocrine neoplasms with 68Ga-DOTA-conjugated somatostatin receptor targeting peptides and 18F-DOPA. Eur J Nucl Med Mol Imaging 44:1588–1601

56. Ambrosini V, Tomassetti P, Castellucci P, Campana D, Montini G, Rubello D et al (2008) Comparison between 68Ga-DOTA-NOC and 18FDOPA PET for the detection of gastro-entero-pancreatic and lung neuroendocrine tumours. Eur J Nucl Med Mol Imaging 35:1431–1438

57. Putzer D, Gabriel M, Henninger B, Kendler D, Uprimny C, Dobrozemsky G et al (2009) Bone metastases in patients with neuroendocrine tumor: 68Ga-DOTA-Tyr3-octreotide PET in comparison to CT and bone scintigraphy. J Nucl Med 50:1214–1221

Hepatocellular Carcinoma

Irene Bargellini, Laura Coletti, and Giulia Lorenzoni

© Springer International Publishing AG 2018
D. Regge, G. Zamboni (eds.), *Hepatobiliary and Pancreatic Cancer*,
Cancer Dissemination Pathways, https://doi.org/10.1007/978-3-319-50296-0_3

3

3.1 Overview

3.1.1 Epidemiology

Hepatocellular carcinoma (HCC) is the most common primary liver tumour and the third leading cause of cancer-related death [1]. Cirrhosis is the most important risk factor, with approximately 80% of HCC cases developing in cirrhotic patients; moreover, HCC represents the leading cause of mortality in patients with cirrhosis [2].

The incidence of HCC is highest in East Asia, sub-Saharan Africa and Melanesia, while in developed regions the incidence is generally low, with the exception of Southern Europe [3].

3.1.2 Risk Factors

In the majority of cases, HCC occurs in cirrhotic livers. The most frequent factors associated with cirrhosis include chronic viral hepatitis (types B and C), alcohol abuse and aflatoxin exposure. Hepatitis virus B (HBV) represents the cause of approximately 70% of HCC cases in Africa and East Asia, whereas in the Western world and in Japan, the majority of cases are related to hepatitis virus C (HCV) infection [3]. In developed countries, however, this scenario is changing. Vaccination and therapy for HBV infection, prevention campaigns for HBV and HCV transmission and newer potent antiviral therapies for HCV are progressively reducing the incidence of HCC related to viral infection, while metabolic disorders associated with obesity, diabetes and fatty liver disease are becoming a more frequent and fearsome risk factor for HCC [4]. Non-alcoholic fatty liver disease (NAFLD) is becoming a major cause of HCC in the United States, and NAFLD-HCC is associated with shorter survival time and more advanced tumour stage [5].

Other factors associated with increased risk of developing HCC include male sex (male to female ratio 2.4), older age (peak incidence around 70 years), cigarette smoking, HIV co-infection, persistent increase in alanine aminotransferase level, increased alfa-fetoprotein (AFP) level and progressive impairment of liver function [6].

3.1.3 Pathology

The majority of HCC develop in the background of liver fibrosis and cirrhosis. In this setting, carcinogenesis is a long-lasting multistep process with progressive malignant transformation from regenerative nodules to low-grade (LGDN) and high-grade (HGDN) dysplastic nodules, early HCC and, finally, overt HCC [7, 8]:

- *Macroregenerative nodules* are benign entities, histologically indistinguishable from the adjacent parenchymal cirrhotic nodules.
- *Dysplastic nodules* are mostly less than 2 cm in diameter and encapsulated and differ from the surrounding liver parenchyma with regard to size, colour, texture and degree of bulging. They are histologically characterized by the presence of portal tracts and:
  - *LGDN*: mild increase in cellularity without architectural atypia;
  - *HGDN*: cytological and architectural atypia insufficient for a diagnosis of malignancy, increased cell density with irregular trabecular pattern and occasional unpaired arteries.
- *Small HCC* are by definition less than 2 cm in size and are divided into two different entities:
  - *Early, vaguely nodular-type HCC*: characterized by indistinct margins with well-differentiated cells and few portal tracts; it is considered as "in situ carcinoma". It can be difficult to differentiate from HGDN; stromal invasion (tumour cells invading the portal tracts or fibrous septa) represents the most reliable morphological feature for differential diagnosis.
  - *Progressed, distinctively nodular-type HCC*: characterized by distinct margins, it presents clear signs of malignancy, with well or moderately differentiated histology, area of steatosis, neoarterialization and possible microvascular invasion (MVI); portal tracts are absent.
- *Overt HCC* typically forms heterogeneous soft masses with areas of haemorrhage or necrosis. Macroscopically, three main patterns have been described. The *nodular or expanding pattern* is more common and characterized by a fibrous capsule and possible satellite nodules (◘ Fig. 3.1). The

infiltrative or massive pattern features large, poorly defined masses with invasive borders (■ Fig. 3.2); the prognosis is poorer. The *diffuse pattern* is less frequent and characterized by small nodules diffused to the entire liver (■ Fig. 3.3).

Histologically, HCC is typically a highly vascularized tumour with different degrees of cellular differentiation (well, moderately and poorly differentiated) based upon the architectural and cytological features.

The most important pathological feature influencing diagnosis and management of HCC is represented by the vascular changes taking place in the process of carcinogenesis. In the malignant nodules, new unpaired arteries develop not accompanied by bile ducts; this process of *arterialization* is directly related to the degree of HCC differentiation, particularly in lesions smaller than 3 cm [9].

Meanwhile, *sinusoidal capillarization* takes place, consisting of transformation of fenestrated hepatic sinusoids into continuous capillaries, coupled with collagenization of the extravascular spaces of Disse and deposition of laminin and basement membranes near the endothelial cells and hepatocytes [9–11]. These vascular changes are the basis of the typical vascular pattern that can be appreciated at contrast-enhanced dynamic imaging.

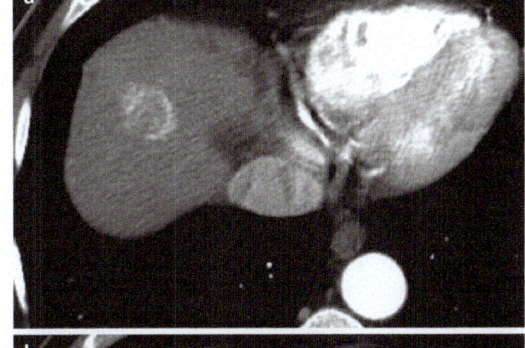

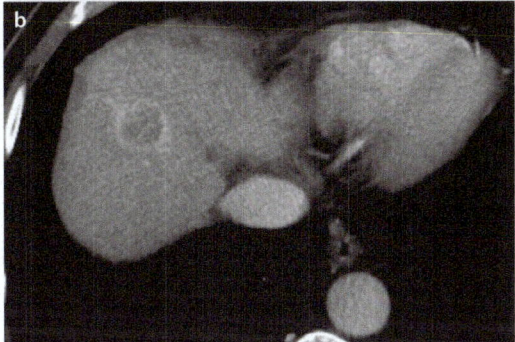

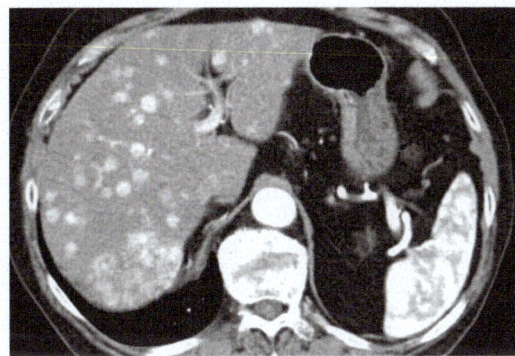

■ **Fig. 3.1** Nodular-type HCC with typical enhancement at CT in late arterial phase **a** and wash-out with tumour capsule in portal venous phase **b**

■ **Fig. 3.3** Diffuse HCC characterized by multiple small arterially enhancing nodules diffused in the entire liver

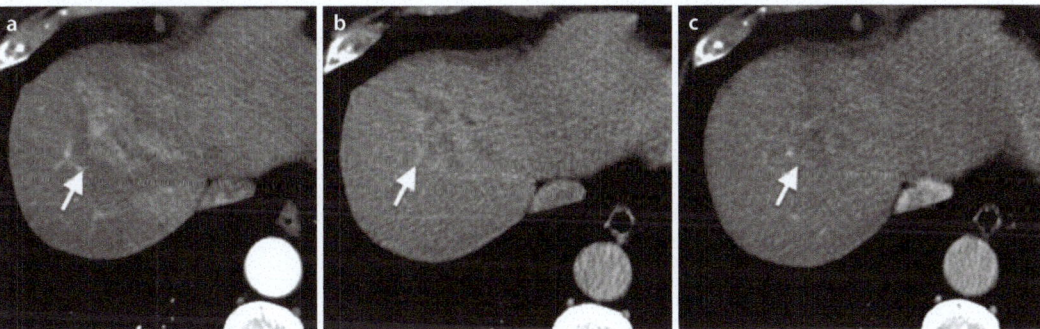

■ **Fig. 3.2** Infiltrative HCC (*arrows*) with poorly defined margins and typical arterial phase wash-in **a** and portal venous **b** and equilibrium **c** phases wash-out

3

Together with these vascular changes, other modifications can be observed and exploited using newer hepatocyte-specific contrast agents, such as a progressive decrease in the number of Kupffer cells and of bile canaliculi [12–16].

A limited number of HCC develop *without liver fibrosis*. These cases have usually a better prognosis, because of the absence of functional liver impairment, allowing more aggressive treatments. For instance, HCC has been described in patients with metabolic syndrome without liver fibrosis. Moreover, some specific tumour variants can develop on normal livers, such as in case of malignant transformation of hepatocellular adenomas and fibrolamellar HCC [17].

3.1.4 Staging

Over the years, numerous staging systems have been proposed for HCC, none of them receiving universal validation and acceptance [18]. Nonetheless, over the last years there has been a general agreement that staging of HCC should take into account not only tumour extension but also the patients' general clinical conditions and liver function.

The *Barcelona Clinic Liver Cancer (BCLC) system* [6, 19, 20] is the most commonly adopted staging modality for HCC in the Western world, and it has been endorsed by the American and

European guidelines [3, 6]. It consists of five different stages, on the basis of tumour extension, patient's performance status [21] and liver function [22] (◻ Tables 3.1, 3.2, and 3.3).

3.1.5 Treatment

Treatment of HCC is strongly dependent on the stage at which the tumour is diagnosed [3, 6].

3.1.5.1 Very Early Stage

In the very early-stage, 5-year survival after curative treatments ranges from 60 to 80%. For several years, resection has been advocated as the first-line treatment in very early-stage HCC. More recent data have shown ablation to be not inferior and more cost-effective than surgery [23, 24], representing today the first-line treatment option in patients not suitable for liver transplantation (LTx) [20].

The role of LTx in this stage of the disease is debated. Some authors have proposed LTx in patients with tumour recurrence [25], while others have proposed to reserve LTx to those patients with pathological evidence of MVI or satellites after first-line resection [26].

3.1.5.2 Early Stage

In the early stage curative treatments are indicated, including LTx, resection and percutaneous ablation. Surgical approaches should represent

◻ **Table 3.1** BCLC (Barcelona Clinic Liver Cancer) staging system [26]

BCLC stage	ECOG PS	Liver function	Tumour stage	First-line treatment
Stage 0 (very early)	0	No portal hypertension, normal bilirubin	Single, <2 cm	Resection Ablation Transplantation
Stage A (early)	0	Child-Pugh A-B	Single; ≤3 tumours, ≤3 cm	
Stage B (intermediate)	0	Child-Pugh A-B	Large multinodular	Transarterial chemoembolization
Stage C (advanced)	1–2	Child-Pugh A-B	Vascular invasion, extrahepatic spread	Sorafenib
Stage D (terminal)	3–4	Child-Pugh C	Any	Best supportive care

Stage 0, A and B: all criteria should be fulfilled
Stages C and D: at least one criterion should be fulfilled
ECOG PS Eastern Cooperative Oncology Group Performance Status

◘ **Table 3.2**   Eastern Cooperative Oncology Group performance status [28]

Stage	
0	Fully active, without restriction
1	Restricted in physically strenuous activity but ambulatory and able to carry out light work
2	Capable of self-care, unable of work activities; up for more than 50% waking hours
3	Limited self-care capacity; confined to bed or chair >50% waking hours
4	Completely disabled; confined to bed or chair
5	Dead

◘ **Table 3.3**   Child-Pugh score [29]

Parameter	1 point	2 points	3 points
Ascites	None	Mild	Moderate to severe
Hepatic encephalopathy	None	Grades I–II	Grades III–IV
Total bilirubin, μmol/L (mg/dL)	<34 (<2)	34–50 (2–3)	>50 (>3)
Serum albumin (g/dL)	>3.5	2.8–3.5	<2.8
Prothrombin time (s)/INR (%)	<4.0/<1.7	4.0–6.0/1.7–2.3	>6.0/>2.3

Class A: 5–6 points
Class B: 7–9 points
Class C: 10–15 points

the first-line options, reaching 60–80% 5-year survival rates [20].

LTx represents the most appealing treatment option, being able to cure both the tumour and the underlying cirrhosis. The Milan criteria (single HCC ≤5 cm or ≤3 nodules each ≤3 cm and no macrovascular invasion on imaging) are used to select patients for LTx [27]. When these criteria

are fulfilled, the 5-year survival rate is approximately 75%. However, these criteria are considered to be restrictive, and expanded selection criteria have been proposed, such as the University of California, San Francisco criteria (single nodule up to 6.5 cm or a maximum of three lesions, none of which larger than 4.5 cm, with a maximum total size less than 8 cm, without vascular invasion or metastases) [28] or the up-to-seven criteria, where seven is the maximum score allowed, summing the size of the largest tumour (in cm) to the total number of tumours [29].

The major limitation for successful transplantation is organ shortage, with patients waiting over 1 year on the waiting list at increased risk for tumour progression and delisting. To avoid progression, resection and ablation, TACE and radioembolization are commonly used to bridge patients to LTx [30, 31].

Early-stage patients excluded from LTx should be considered for *resection*, particularly in the presence of single lesion and normal bilirubin, without signs of portal hypertension [3, 6, 20].

Ablation represents the first-line approach in patients excluded from surgery; radiofrequency (RF) ablation is the most frequently adopted technique, although microwave ablation is becoming a strong competitor. Tumour location, size and number may limit the indications for percutaneous ablation. In fact, the success of ablation is lower when more than two nodules are treated and in tumours >3 cm in size and in perivascular location [32]. Larger tumours could benefit from sequential treatments by TACE and ablation [33], when surgery is contraindicated.

Tumour recurrence after ablation or resection remains a matter of concern. In fact, 50–80% of patients will experience recurrence within 5 years after resection and the majority within 2 years [34]. Likewise, 3-year cumulative recurrence rates of about 50% are reported after RF ablation [35, 36]. Predictors of recurrence are tumour size, multifocality, vascular invasion and poor differentiation. Up to now, adjuvant treatments have failed in reducing the risk of recurrence [37].

3.1.5.3 Intermediate Stage

TACE represents the first-line treatment modality in intermediate-stage HCC patients, with reported median survival of around 20 months [38–40], reaching 40 months in well-selected patients [41–43].

3

The combination of TACE and molecular target agents (sorafenib and brivanib) has not proven to improve clinical outcomes [44, 45].

Other treatment options in the selected intermediate-stage patients include combined TACE and ablation, radioembolization with Yttrium-90 labelled spheres (Y90-RE) and resection and LTx after successful tumour downstaging (defined as the reduction of the tumour burden to meet acceptable criteria, based on expected survival after LTx that should be equal to that of patients who meet transplant criteria without downstaging) [33, 46–50].

3.1.5.4 Advanced Stage

According to guidelines, sorafenib represents the first-line treatment option in advanced-stage HCC [3, 6, 20], able to increase survival and time to progression [51, 52].

Numerous other trials have investigated the role of other molecular-targeted agents, all of them failing in demonstrating additional benefits compared to sorafenib or placebo in first- and second-line systemic treatments. Only recently, the results of the phase III RESORCE trial have been presented showing that, compared to placebo, regorafenib improves overall survival in patients progressing after treatment with sorafenib [53]. Thus, a second-line treatment is today available in selected patients.

Y90-RE represents another appealing treatment option in advanced-stage HCC, particularly in patients with limited portal vein tumour thrombosis, achieving highly competitive survival rates compared to sorafenib, with lower toxicities [54–56]. Prospective, multicentre, randomized trials are ongoing to evaluate results of Y90-RE in comparison to TACE or sorafenib or in combination with sorafenib.

Finally, in highly selected patients with limited macrovascular tumour invasion and preserved liver function, *resection* has been proposed showing excellent long-term survival rates [57, 58].

3.1.6 Prognosis

Prognosis largely depends on the stage at which the tumour is detected. Patients presenting with very advanced HCC are considered untreatable and will die within 3–6 months [3]. However, early detection by surveillance programmes and refinements of treatments for viral infection, liver cirrhosis and tumours have contributed to the improvement of prognosis over the last 15 years [4].

3.2 HCC: Imaging Features and Prognosis

Due to the characteristics of vascular changes occurring in the process of carcinogenesis, HCC can be reliably diagnosed by cross-sectional imaging. In fact, non-invasive diagnosis of HCC is possible in patients with liver cirrhosis when a nodule >1 cm in diameter is detected at dynamic contrast-enhanced computed tomography (CT) and/or magnetic resonance imaging (MRI), with arterial hyper-enhancement (wash-in) and portal venous or delayed phase hypo-enhancement (wash-out) (◘ Fig. 3.1) [3, 6, 20]. These imaging features enable diagnosis of HCC with almost 100% specificity and positive predictive value.

Besides this typical vascular pattern, imaging enables the identification of additional tumoural features that may represent prognostic factors related to tumour dissemination and patient survival, such as *tumour size, intratumoural fat, mosaic architecture, fibrous capsule, corona enhancement* and *multifocality* [11].

3.2.1 Tumour Size

Compared to small lesions, *large HCCs* (>2 cm) tend to have a higher histologic grade and a more aggressive biologic behaviour, increasing the risk for vascular invasion and extrahepatic tumour metastasis. For these reasons, it is clinically important to identify small HCCs prior to their growth beyond 2 cm.

3.2.2 Intralesional Fat

Intralesional fatty change occurs during hepatocarcinogenesis in approximately 10% of HCCs [59]. It has been reported that patients with lesions showing intratumoural fat may have better prognosis, with longer time to tumour progression and reduced risk of metastasis. A possible explanation is that intralesional fat is a typical feature of early and well-differentiated HCC, not described in poorly differentiated lesions. MRI with chemical shift (in- and opposed-phase) sequences represents a simple, highly sensitive and specific method to demonstrate intratumoural fatty infiltration (▣ Fig. 3.4).

3.2.3 Mosaic Architecture

Mosaic architecture is the presence of intratumoural heterogeneity caused by fibrotic septa, necrosis, haemorrhage, copper deposition and fatty infiltration (▣ Fig. 3.5) [11]. This feature is

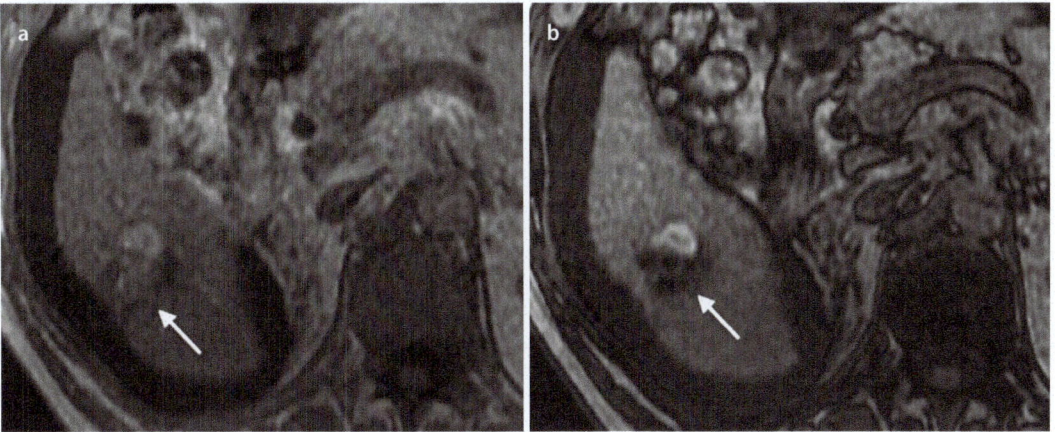

▣ **Fig. 3.4** Axial MRI with chemical shift (in-phase, **a**; opposed-phase, **b**) demonstrating intratumoural fatty infiltration (*arrows*)

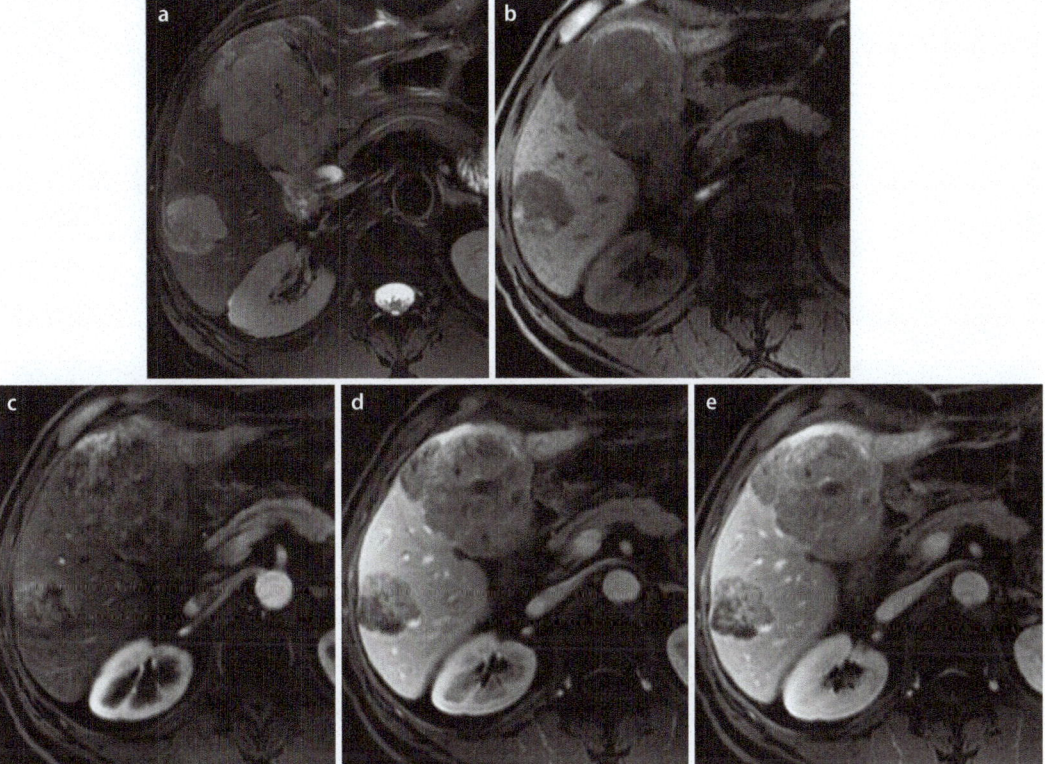

▣ **Fig. 3.5** Axial MRI (T2-weighted, **a** T1-weighted, **b** arterial phase, **c** portal venous phase, **d** equilibrium phase, **e**) demonstrating two large HCC with mosaic architecture

more frequently observed in large HCCs. Mosaic architecture is unusual in tumours other than HCC; therefore, it has been included among the ancillary features favouring the diagnosis of HCC in the recent LI-RADS (Liver Imaging Reporting and Data System) proposed by the American College of Radiology [60, 61]. Mosaic architecture is considered an unfavourable prognostic sign, associated with increased risk of postsurgical recurrence [62].

3.2.4 Tumour Capsule

Tumour capsule can be appreciated in 60–80% of HCC nodules and has been listed among the features enabling HCC diagnosis in the LI-RADS (◘ Fig. 3.1) [60]. Although a tumour capsule is more frequently described in lesions larger than 2 cm, it represents a favourable prognostic factor compared to nodules of similar grade and

size without capsule or with disrupted capsule [63, 64]. This may be due to the barrier effect of the fibrous capsule that inhibits HCC dissemination.

3.2.5 Corona Enhancement

Corona enhancement is related to the enhancement of the venous drainage in the peritumoural parenchyma. In progressed HCCs, the portal venules draining the tumour communicate with the sinusoids in the peritumoural parenchyma, determining corona-shaped perinodular enhancement a few seconds after the tumoural enhancement [11]. While tumour capsule appears as a progressively enhancing rim in portal venous and delayed phases (◘ Fig. 3.1), corona enhancement is appreciated in the late arterial or early venous phases and fades in the subsequent phases (◘ Fig. 3.6). The presence of large [65] or irregular

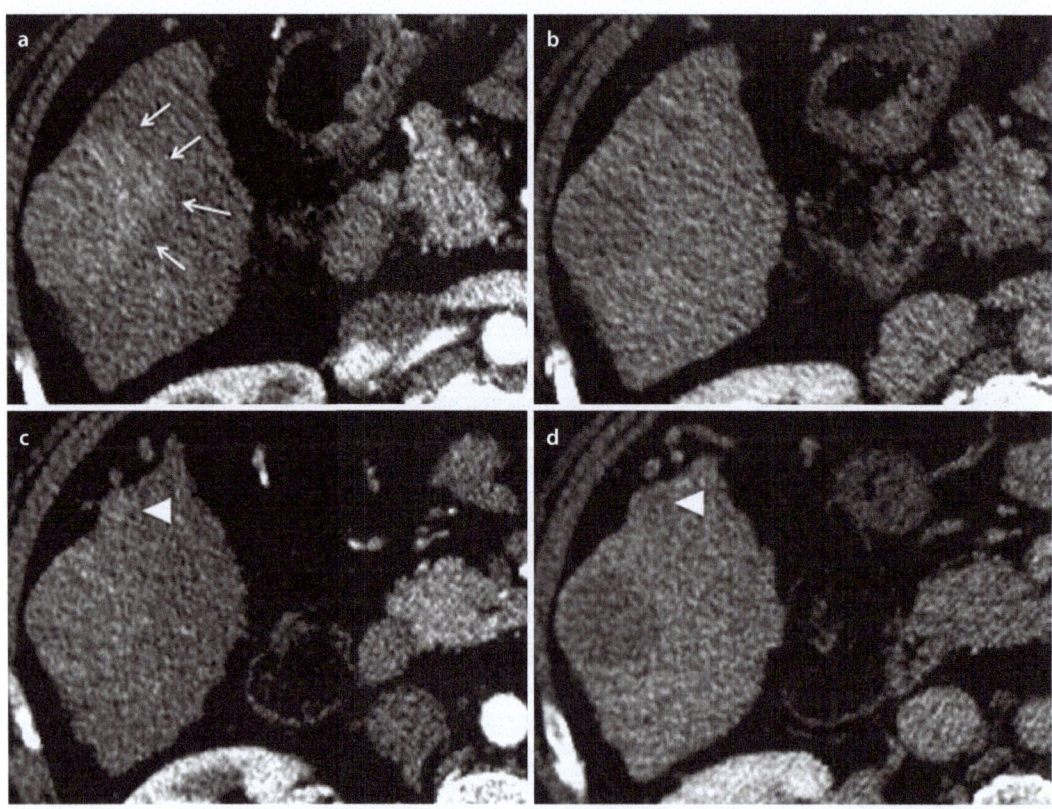

◘ Fig. 3.6 Axial CT (late arterial phase, **a** and **c**; equilibrium phase, **b** and **d**) showing HCC with corona enhancement in late arterial phase (**a**, *arrows*) disappear-ing in equilibrium phase **b**; a small satellite nodule is visible (**c** and **d**, *arrowheads*)

and/or distorted [66] corona enhancement may predict MVI and can indicate a higher risk for local recurrence after resection or ablation [67]. Thus, some authors recommend including the corona enhancement areas within the margins of resection or ablation [67].

3.2.6 Multifocality

Multifocal tumours are associated with poorer prognosis and reduced therapeutic chances. They are either multiple independent HCCs arising simultaneously (multicentric HCC) or intrahepatic metastases from a primary HCC

(■ Fig. 3.7) [68]. Multicentric HCC is expected to show a more favourable biological behaviour, while metastatic HCC is associated with earlier recurrences and poorer prognosis. Therefore, differentiation is of major importance. In general, multicentric tumours present as small, uniform nodules in different segments (■ Fig. 3.8), and histologically they can show different features, including variable grades of differentiation, as a representation of the multistep carcinogenesis. As opposite, metastatic HCCs can be visualized as small satellites surrounding a larger lesion and are usually moderately to poorly differentiated, with no evidence of multistep carcinogenesis (■ Fig. 3.9) [8, 11, 69].

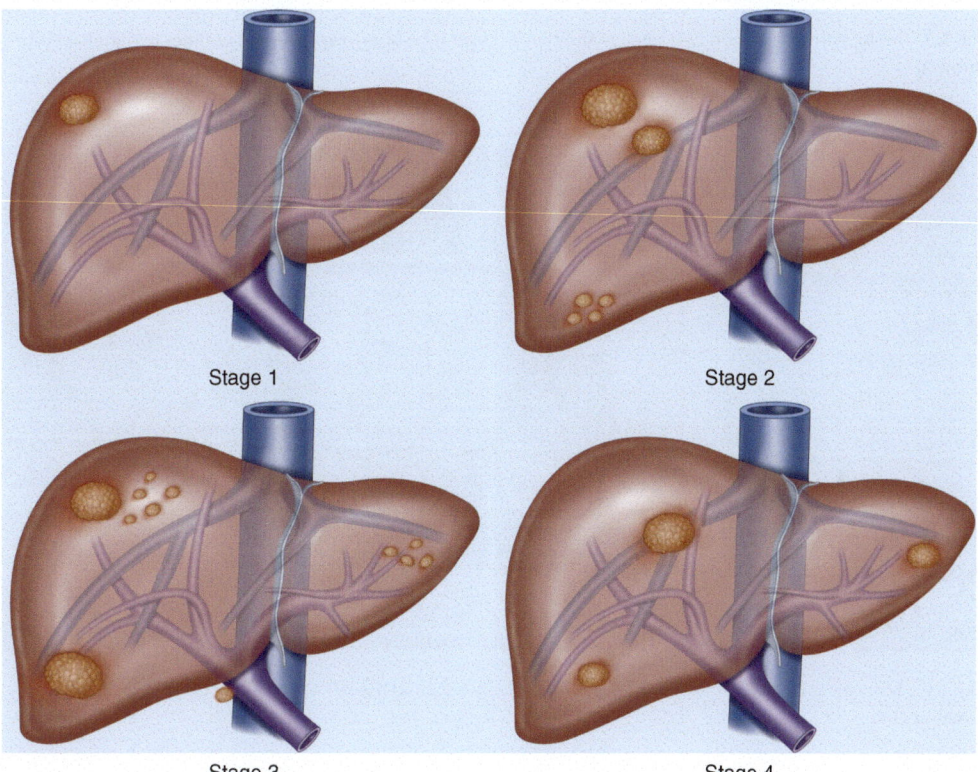

Stage 1

Stage 2

Stage 3

Stage 4

■ **Fig. 3.7** Intrahepatic dissemination according to TNM classification:

■ **Stage 1:** solitary, <2 cm without vascular invasion

■ – **Stage 2:** solitary, <2 cm with vascular invasion; solitary, >2 cm or multiple, one lobe <2 cm without vascular invasion

■ – **Stage 3:** solitary, >2 cm with vascular invasion; multiple, one lobe <2 cm with vascular invasion; multiple, one lobe >2 cm without vascular invasion

■ – **Stage 4:** multiple, > one lobe and/or invasion of major branch of portal or hepatic veins

3

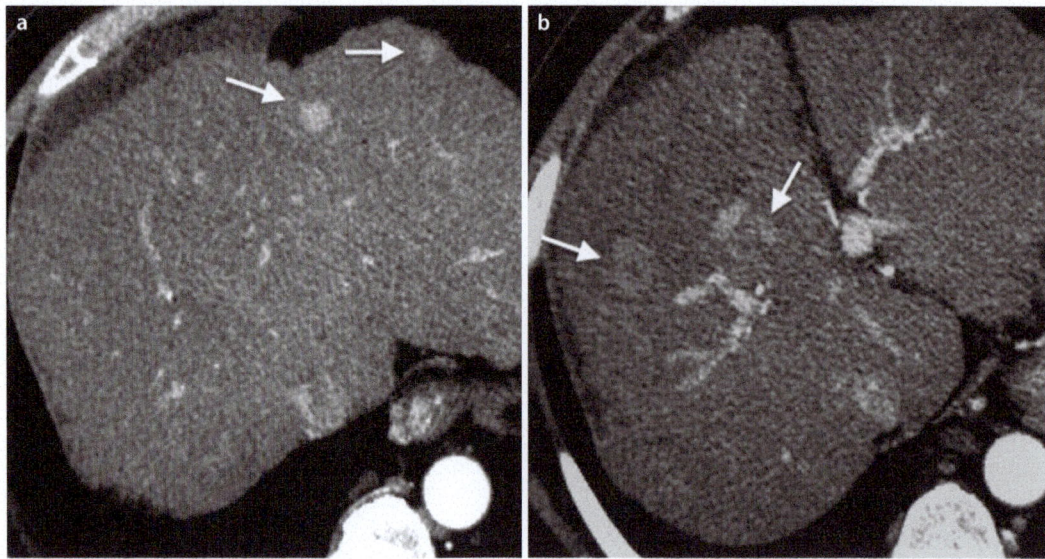

▪ **Fig. 3.8** Multicentric HCC, with two small nodules in left liver lobe (**a**, *arrows*) and two nodules in right liver lobe (**b**, *arrows*)

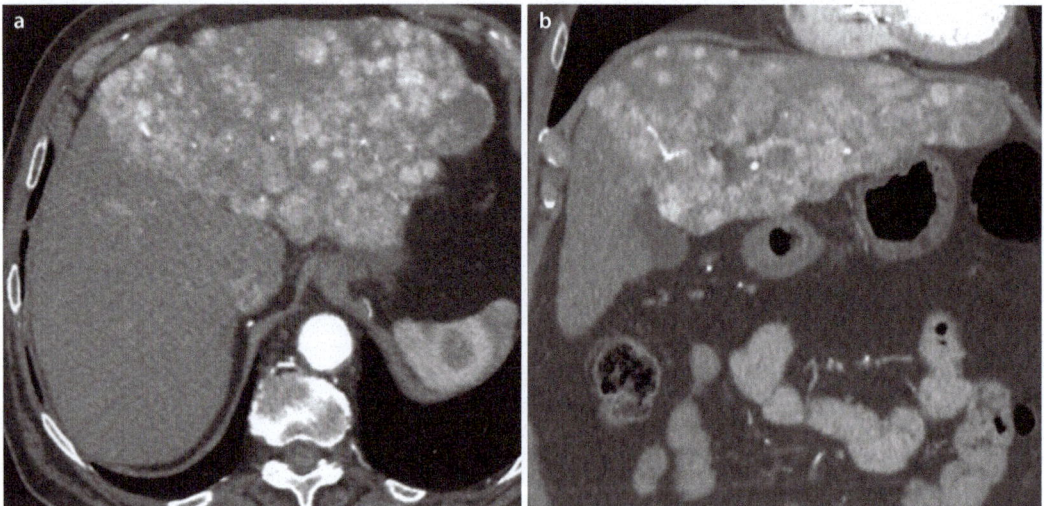

▪ **Fig. 3.9** Metastatic HCC with multiple nodules extensively invading the left hepatic lobe (axial scan, **a**; coronal reformation, **b**)

3.3 HCC: Intrahepatic Dissemination

In the early stages, the majority of HCC grow as encapsulated or expanding masses. As the tumour enlarges, it infiltrates the surrounding liver parenchyma forming satellite nodules, which by definition should be located within 2 cm from the main tumour and should be ≤2 cm in size (▪ Fig. 3.10).

3.3.1 Microvascular Invasion

The most frequent pathway of HCC dissemination is through the venous circulation, starting from *MVI*. This is defined as the histological identification of tumour emboli within the vascular spaces rimmed by endothelium [8], it is responsible for intrahepatic and extrahepatic metastasis, as well as portal and hepatic vein macrovascular invasion, and it is related to

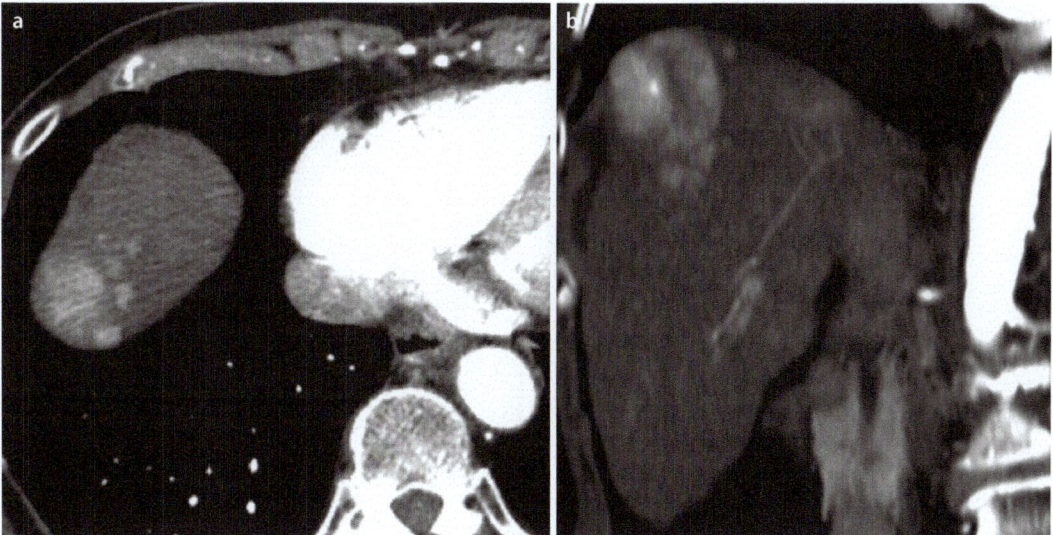

◘ Fig. 3.10   Axial **a** and oblique coronal views **b** showing a larger lesion surrounded by multiple small satellite nodules

tumour size, being observed in over 50% of larger HCC. MVI cannot be reliable detected at imaging. However, some imaging features are reported to be closely related to increased risk of MVI, such as the presence of more than three nodules, the tumour size exceeding 3 cm [70], the detection of corona enhancement [11, 66], a lower apparent diffusion coefficient (ADC) measured with diffusion-weighted MR imaging [70] and 18F-fluorodeoxyglucose (FDG) uptake [71] at positron emission tomography (PET)/CT [72].

More recently, a computed tomography radiogenomic biomarker has been derived from a 91-gene HCC "venous invasion" gene expression signature that is able to predict MVI and prognosis in HCC surgical candidates [73]. This biomarker considers several features, such as tumour size, tumour-to-liver interface, heterogeneity, the presence of internal arteries and enhancement pattern [74].

3.3.2 Intrahepatic Metastases

Intrahepatic metastases develop by two different pathways [67, 75]. Tumour cells may enter the portal venules draining from the primary tumour and spread into the surrounding parenchyma generating satellite nodules, as described above. Alternatively, tumour cells may enter directly into the systemic circulation, generating metastatic

nodules outside the drainage area, including other segments and the contralateral lobe.

As already mentioned, prognosis of patients with intrahepatic metastasis from HCC is poorer compared to patients with multicentric HCC [69], since the tumour is usually poorly differentiated, has a more aggressive biological behaviour and has already invaded the systemic circulation.

3.3.3 Macroscopic Vascular Invasion

Vascular invasion involves more frequently the portal venous system than the hepatic veins and is more common in large and poorly differentiated HCC [75]. Macrovascular invasion distinguishes HCC from metastatic neoplasms that rarely invade the intrahepatic vessels.

Macroscopic portal vein vascular invasion (PVI) usually occurs during tumour enlargement involving the contiguous portal vein branches. Thus, besides tumour size, tumour location in respect to the portal vein branches represents an important risk factor (◘ Fig. 3.11). Diagnosis of PVI is based on the identification of enlarged portal vein branches with solid component showing hyper-enhancement in the late arterial phase and wash-out in the portal venous and/or equilibrium phases at CT, MRI and contrast-enhanced ultrasound (◘ Fig. 3.12). However, differentiating PVI from bland thrombosis may be challenging (◘ Fig. 3.13) [76], and additional imaging

3

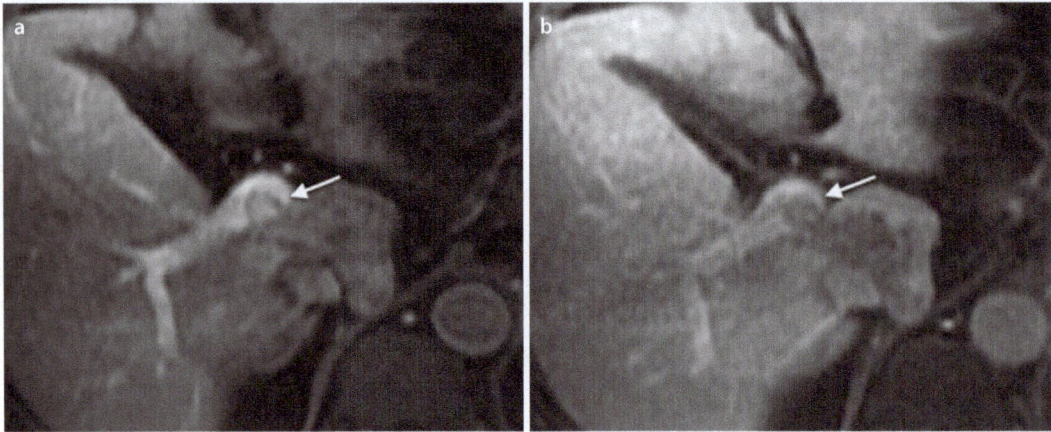

◘ **Fig. 3.11** Axial MRI in late arterial **a** and portal venous phases **b** showing HCC in segment 1 invading the main portal trunk (*arrows*)

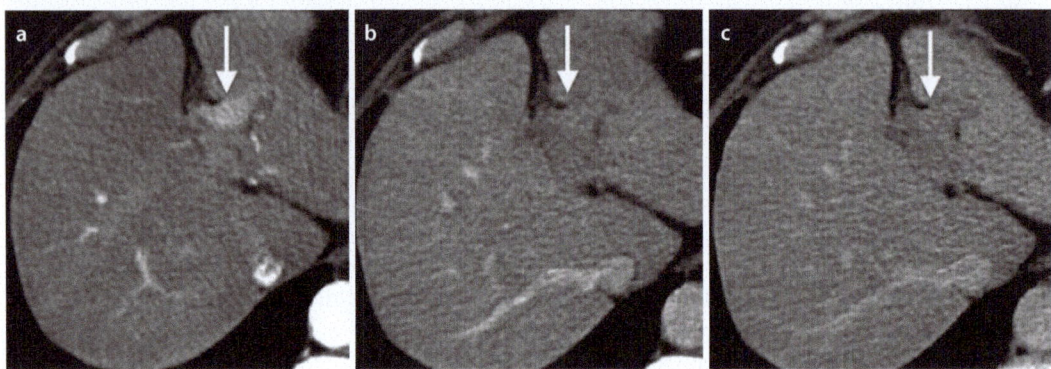

◘ **Fig. 3.12** Macroscopic vascular invasion of left portal branch (*arrows*), with arterial phase wash-in **a** and portal venous **b** and equilibrium phase **c** wash-out

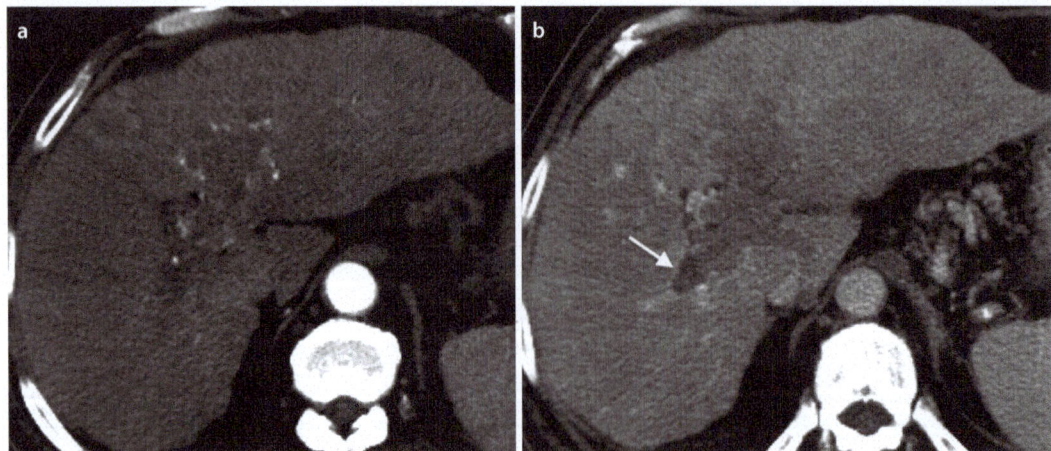

◘ **Fig. 3.13** Macroscopic vascular invasion of left, right and main portal branches (late arterial phase), **a** portal venous phase, **b**, with limited bland thrombosis in the right portal branch (**b**, *arrow*)

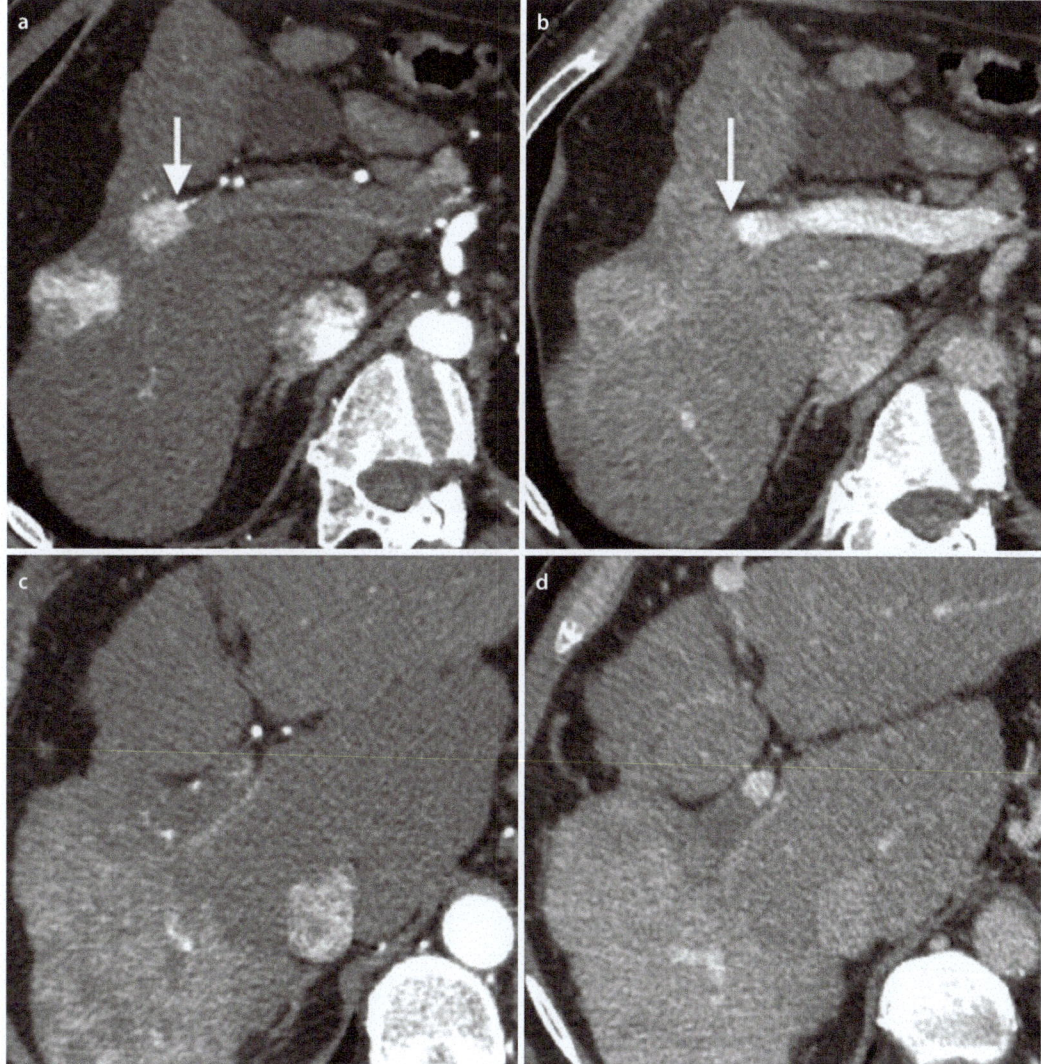

🔲 **Fig. 3.14** Oblique CT reformations in late arterial **a** and portal venous **b** phases show macroscopic HCC invasion of the segmental portal branch for segment 5 (*arrows*). Three months after Y90-RE complete lesion devascularisation is observed (late arterial phase, **a**; portal venous phase, **b**)

parameters have been proposed, such as intermediate signal intensity in T2-weighted MR images [77], iodine mapping obtained from dual-energy CT [78] and ADC measurement on DWI [79].

The extent of PVI impacts patients' prognosis. In fact, several studies have reported significantly higher survival rates in patients with segmental or sectorial PVI compared to patients with tumour thrombus extending to the left or right main portal vein, the main trunk or even beyond [54, 55, 80, 81]. These findings suggest that minor PVI (limited to sectorial/segmental branches) should be considered for more aggressive treatments, such as resection, Y90-RE (🔲 Fig. 3.14)

and TACE, even combined with percutaneous ablation [54, 55, 57, 58, 82, 83]. Indeed, the reported median survival of advanced HCC patients after resection (27.8 months) [82], drug-eluting bead TACE (13.5 months) [83] or Y90-RE (13.0 months) [54] seems to be at least comparable to or even longer than the median survival reported after sorafenib alone (10.7 months in the SHARP trial and 6.5 months in the Asia Pacific Study) [51, 52].

Macroscopic hepatic vein vascular invasion (HVI) is less frequent than PVI (🔲 Fig. 3.15). In HVI, the thrombus can extend into the inferior vena cava (IVC) leading to the formation of

3

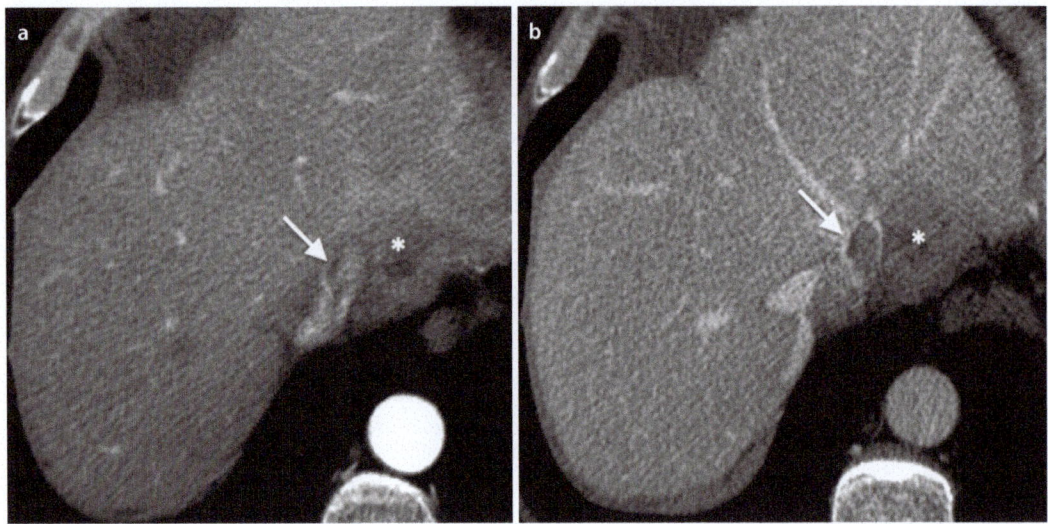

◼ **Fig. 3.15** Infiltrative HCC (*asterisk*) with macroscopic invasion of left hepatic vein (*arrows*; late arterial phase, **a**; portal venous phase, **b**)

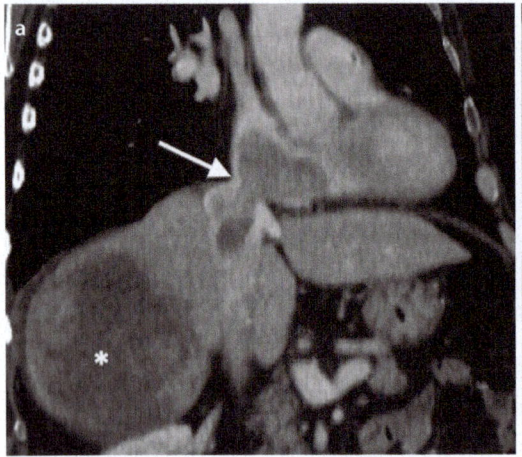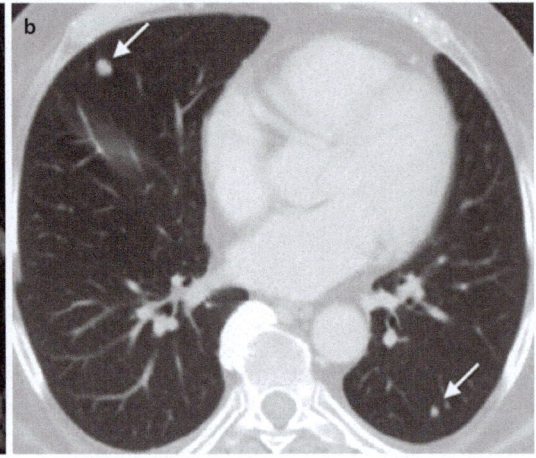

◼ **Fig. 3.16** Coronal oblique CT reformation **a** showing large HCC in the right hepatic lobe invading the right hepatic vein, inferior vena cava and right

atrium (*arrow*) and associated with intrapulmonary dissemination (**b**, *arrows*)

thrombi in the right atrium, intrapulmonary dissemination (◼ Fig. 3.16), pulmonary embolism or even sudden death, thus leading to a poorer prognosis compared to PVI, particularly when the thrombosis extends into the IVC [84]. As for PVI, although the standard of care should be sorafenib according to European and American guidelines [3, 6], more aggressive treatments, including TACE, Y90-RE and surgery, have been proposed in selected patients, with promising clinical outcomes [54, 55, 57, 84, 85].

3.3.4 Biliary Tumour Thrombus

A relatively rare pathway of HCC dissemination is through the biliary tree, with a reported incidence of 0.53–12.9% in autopsy and surgical specimens [86].

Biliary tumour thrombus (BTT) is defined as the macroscopic or microscopic identification of tumour emboli within the bile ducts, it can be responsible for jaundice and biliary enlargement [87] and it is frequently related to tumour size and differentiation. Usually, it is detected as a

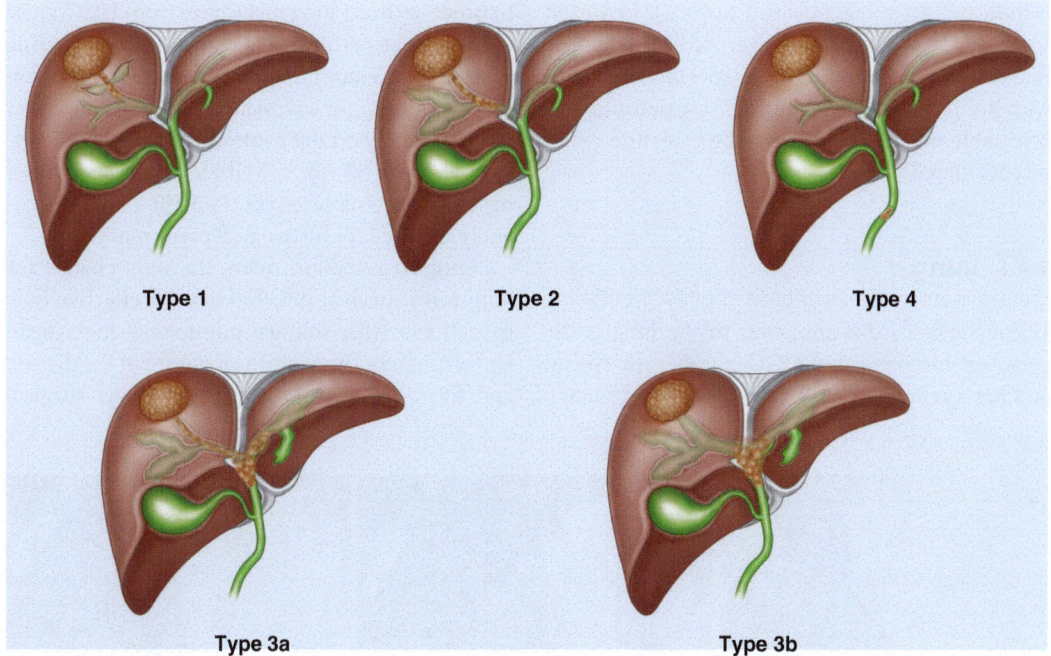

Type 1   Type 2   Type 4

Type 3a   Type 3b

Fig. 3.17 Biliary tumour thrombus classification [88]: type 1, involving the second-order intrahepatic duct; type 2, involving the first-order intrahepatic duct; type 3a, extending to the hepatic confluence; type 3b, growing in the common hepatic duct; type 4, dislodged within the common hepatic duct

free-floating thrombus or as an extended invasion within dilated bile ducts [87]; however, in some cases BTT cannot be reliable detected at imaging.

HCC with BTT is classified according to the location of BTT, as proposed by Ueda et al. [88]: type 1, involving the second-order intrahepatic duct; type 2, involving the first-order intrahepatic duct; type 3a, extending to the hepatic confluence; type 3b, implanted tumour growing in the common hepatic duct; and type 4, dislodged BTT within the common hepatic duct (Fig. 3.17).

BTT is associated with poorer prognosis, due to a more aggressive biological behaviour and the frequent association with vascular invasion and poor tumour differentiation [86]. In HCC with BTT, surgical treatment is recommended whenever possible to improve long-term survival [86–88].

3.4 HCC: Extrahepatic Metastasis

Due to improvements in diagnostic modalities and prolonged survival, extrahepatic metastasis (EM) are today more frequently observed in patients with HCC.

In the BCLC staging system, patients with EM are considered equal to patients with macroscopic vascular invasion. However, with the exception of patients with regional nodal metastasis, several studies reported poorer survival in patients with EM compared to patients with PVI and no EM [54, 55, 80]. Thus, these two entities should be considered separately from a prognostic point of view [58, 80].

Cause of death in HCC patients with EM is generally related to progression of intrahepatic disease and not to the metastatic tumour spread, indicating the importance of controlling intrahepatic tumours even in HCC patients with EM. However, the presence of EM itself is an indicator of the primary tumour's aggressiveness with limited response to locoregional treatments [89].

Most studies report lungs (47%) and abdominal lymph nodes (45%) as the most frequent sites of extrahepatic disease, but bones (37%) and adrenal glands (12%) can also be involved [90–92]. Rarely, HCC metastases may be found in the skin, brain, muscles, kidney, pancreas and ovary.

Several imaging technique as CT, MRI, radionuclide bone scanning and 18F-FDG PET/CT can be used for identification of EM. In HCC patients with high AFP levels, lung CT and radionuclide bone scanning are usually recommended to rule out EM.

As for the other conditions of advanced-stage HCC, according to Western guidelines sorafenib is indicated for patients with EM [3, 6]. However, sorafenib is a disease stabilizer, with a response rate lower than 9%. Thus, in specific situations with limited intrahepatic tumour burden and few, resectable metastases, resection or ablation could be considered [93–95].

3.4.1 Lung

Haematogenous dissemination to the lung is the prevalent mechanism of HCC extrahepatic spread and has a reported prevalence of 18–60% [90, 91].

In order to detect lung metastases from HCC, chest CT should be performed at regular intervals during routine follow-up. Lung metastasis present as soft tissue nodules, preferentially located in the lower lobes, and may exhibit contrast enhancement in the arterial phase (◘ Fig. 3.18) [92]. Pleural metastases have also been reported (◘ Fig. 3.19). Biopsy is generally required for histological confirmation.

Surgical resection offers the only chance for long-term survival [96, 97], but it is effective only in patients with solitary pulmonary metastasis. Unfortunately, the multifocal nature of the disease and the poor hepatic reserve limit the surgical

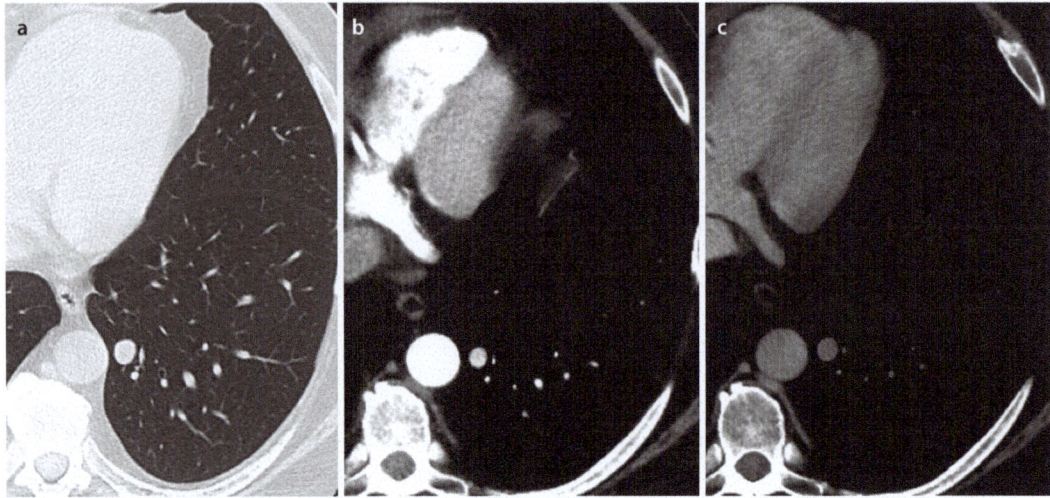

◘ **Fig. 3.18** Lung metastasis **a**, with arterial enhancement **b** and equilibrium phase **c** wash-out

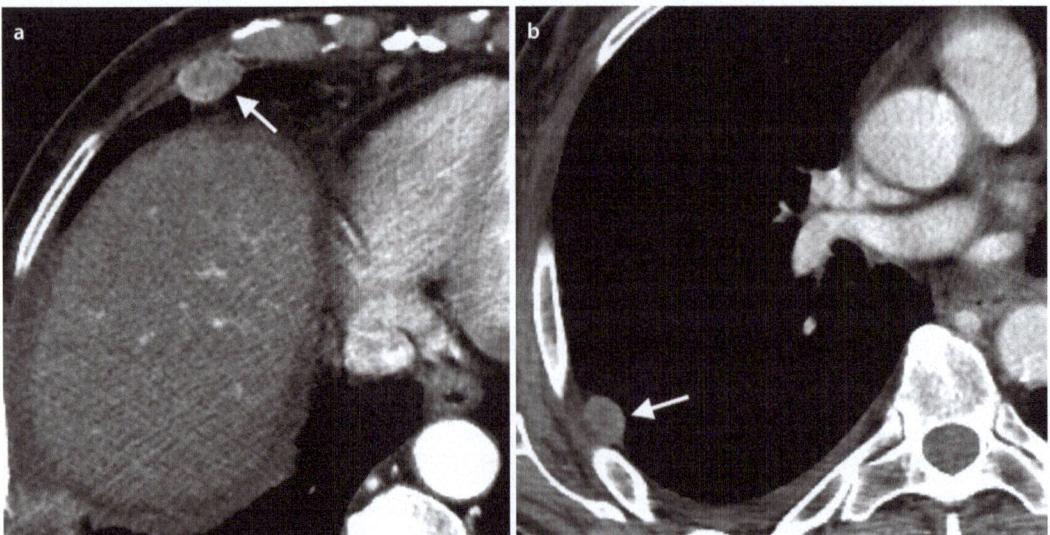

◘ **Fig. 3.19** Pleural metastasis with typical arterial enhancement in middle **a** and lower right **b** lobes (*arrows*)

options. Thus, minimally invasive alterative options have been proposed, such as percutaneous ablation and brachytherapy, frequently combined with systemic chemotherapy. A multicentre study from Hiraki et al. demonstrated an overall survival rate after RF ablation for HCC pulmonary metastases of 87% at 1 year and 57% at 3 years [98].

3.4.2 Lymph Nodes

Lymph nodes are the second most common site of metastasis after lungs, with a reported frequency of 27–42% [99, 100]. More frequently, the lymphatic spread follows the descending deep lymphatic networks along the portal vein, that involve the hilar hepatic lymph nodes (■ Fig. 3.20), from where cells gain access to the celiac nodes and then to the intestinal nodes. Another possible pathway of dissemination involves the ascending deep network, involving the nodes close to inferior vena cava and reaching the mediastinum (■ Fig. 3.21). At times, the lymphatic spread may engage the superficial lymphatic networks, consisting in four different areas: the lateral and medial anterior diaphragmatic groups draining into the pericardiac and subxiphoid nodes, the falciform ligament draining into the anterior abdominal wall and the epigastric and the subxiphoid nodes that drain into the internal mammary nodes (■ Fig. 3.22).

As opposite to other neoplasms, the size of the lymph nodes (1.5–4 cm) is not a reliable criterion

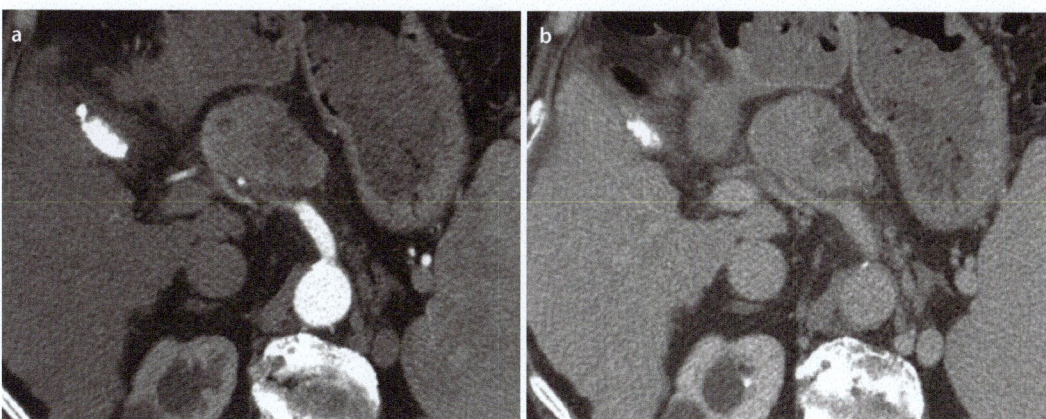

■ **Fig. 3.20**   Large, inhomogeneously enhancing hepatic lymph node metastasis with inhomogeneous mild arterial enhancement **a** and venous hypoattenuation **b**

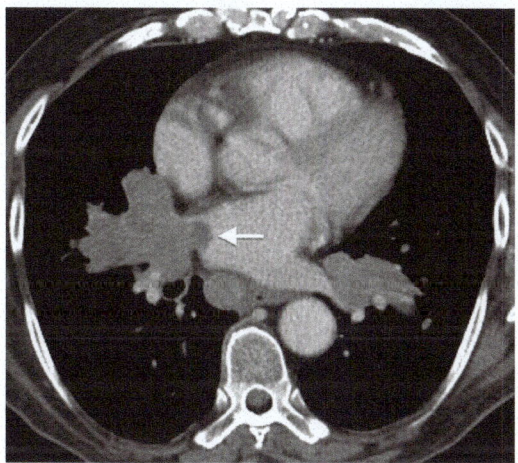

■ **Fig. 3.21**   Multiple extensive mediastinal nodal metastases with thrombus in the right pulmonary vein (*arrow*)

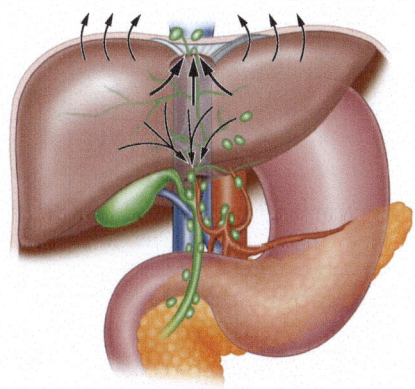

■ **Fig. 3.22**   Patterns of lymphatic dissemination

3

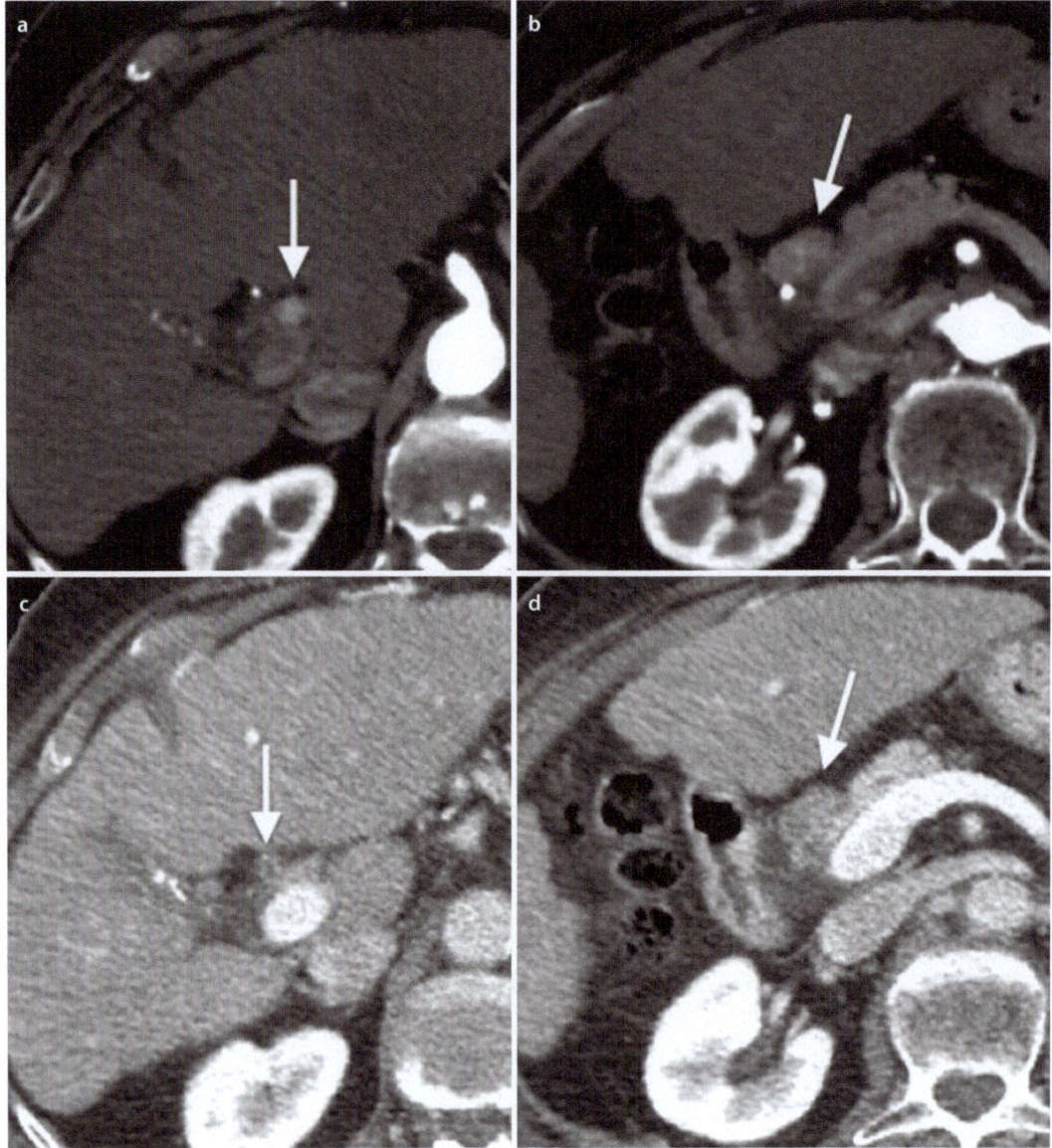

Fig. 3.23 Small regional lymph node metastases showing arterial enhancement (**a**, **b**; *arrows*) and portal venous wash-out (**c**, **d**; *arrows*)

for malignancy [100], since it is well known that cirrhotic patients have benign enlarged lymph nodes. The most useful criterion for diagnosis of malignancy is represented by the contrast enhancement in the arterial phase, as for the primary tumour (■ Fig. 3.23).

Compared to distant EM, patients with regional nodal metastasis have a better prognosis. Thus, although according to guidelines, sorafenib is the standard of care for patients with lymph node metastases, locoregional treatments of the primary tumour should be considered in patients with limited regional nodal involvement, whenever possible, to control the intrahepatic disease. Accordingly, resection and ablation of regional metastasis have been described in selected cases [101, 102].

3.4.3 Bone

The most frequent site of bone metastases is the vertebra (■ Fig. 3.24), possibly because of cell dissemination through the portal vein-vertebral vein

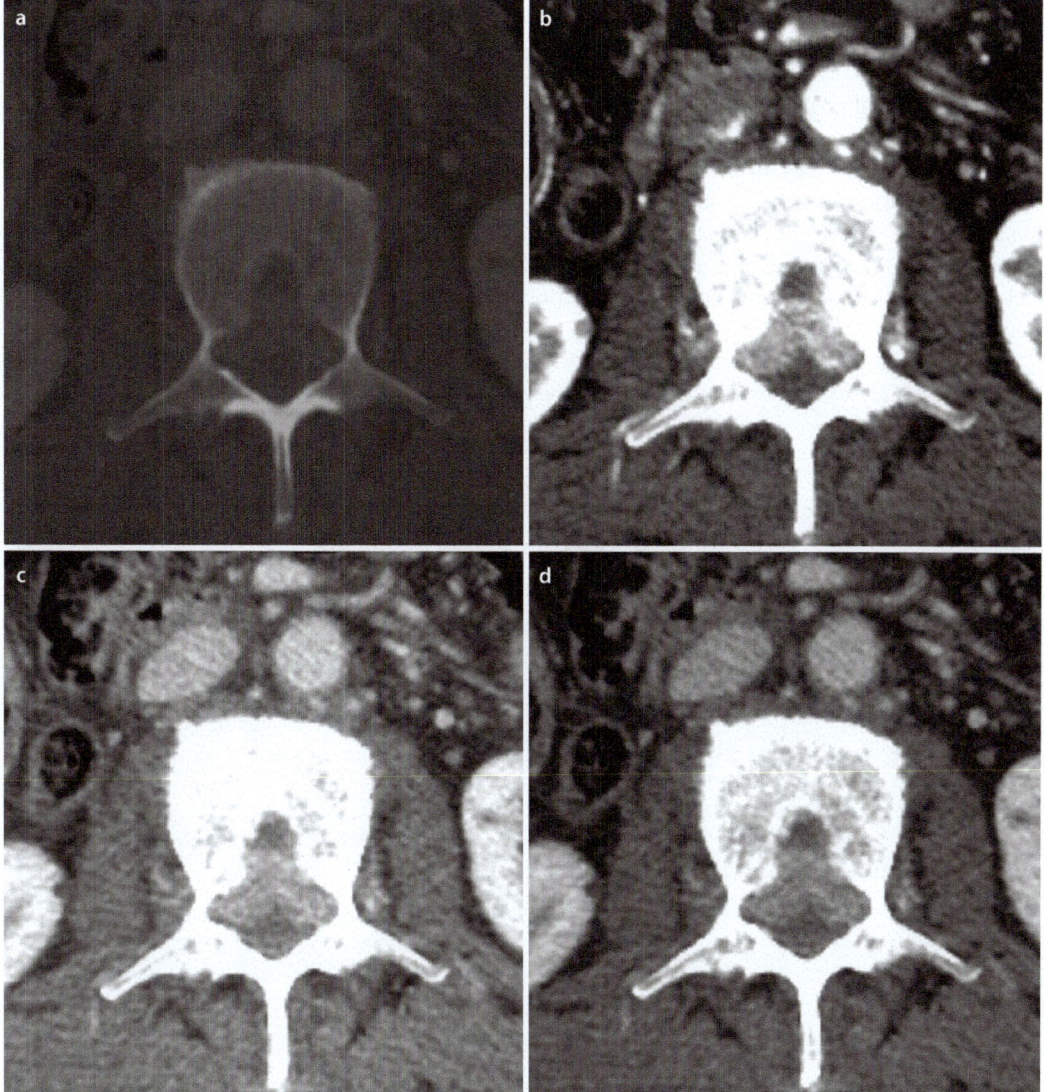

■ **Fig. 3.24**   Metastasis of second lumbar vertebra with large lytic area **a** and solid tissue with typical wash-in **b** and wash-out **c, d**

plexuses due to the presence of portal thrombus and/or portal hypertension, followed by pelvis and ribs [103]. Bone metastases are frequently multiple and invariably lytic. When sufficiently large, the lesion shows solid content, with expanding growth and arterial enhancement (■ Fig. 3.24).

The poor quality life of patients with bone metastasis is due to pain, pathological fractures and reduced mobility. Radiotherapy and medical therapy are used to control pain [104]. However, tumour relapse and adverse events (nausea, loss of appetite, diarrhoea and radiodermatitis) after radiotherapy are frequent. Recently, RF ablation

has been proposed [105]. Surgical or percutaneous stabilization of lytic lesions is indicated to improve quality of life, and it can be combined with RF ablation or preoperative arterial embolization to prevent tumour dissemination and reduce intraoperative blood loss [106].

3.4.4 Adrenal Glands

Adrenal metastases are found in up to 8–17% of metastatic cases [91]. Adrenal spread may follow a random pattern in terms of laterality: one or both adrenal glands can be involved, with the right and left equally affected.

Similar to the problem of differentiating benign from malignant lymphadenopathy, the presence of an enlarged adrenal mass does not always imply malignancy. Adrenal adenomas are a more common cause of an enlarged adrenal gland, even in cancer patients. Differential diagnosis is possible when enhancement in the arterial phase is visualized indicating a metastatic mass (◘ Fig. 3.25).

Several treatment strategies have been proposed for HCC adrenal metastases, including surgery (◘ Fig. 3.26), percutaneous ablation, TACE and radiotherapy [107–110].

3.4.5 Other Metastatic Sites

In addition to haematogenous and lymphatic dissemination, HCC can directly infiltrate contiguous structures, such as the diaphragm (◘ Fig. 3.27), the falciform ligament and the abdominal wall (◘ Figs. 3.28 and 3.29) [92]. Peritoneum dissemination is a rare condition (◘ Fig. 3.30).

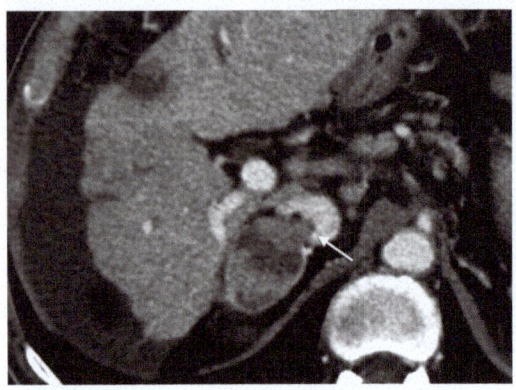

◘ **Fig. 3.25** Right adrenal metastasis invading the inferior vena cava (*arrow*)

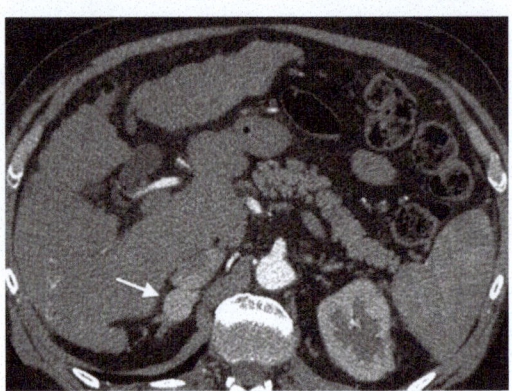

◘ **Fig. 3.26** Small, bioptically proven right adrenal metastasis (*arrow*); adrenalectomy was performed

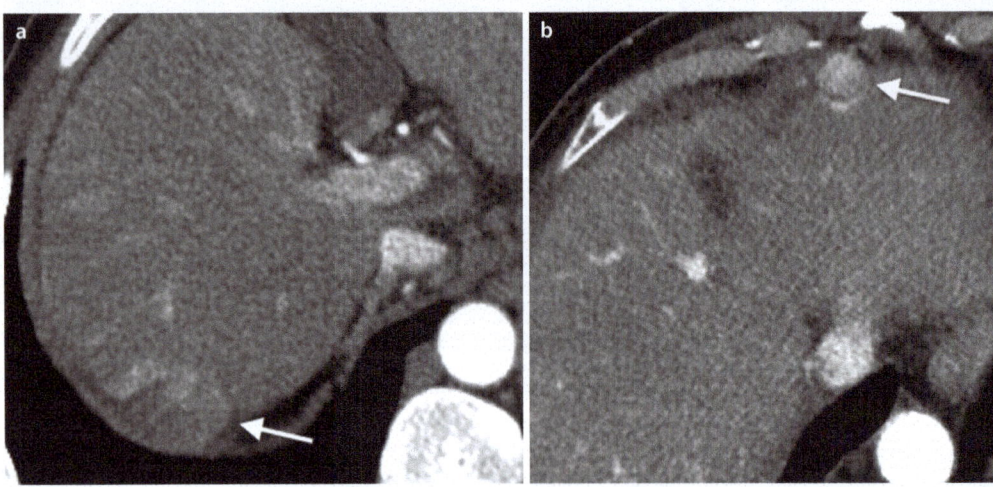

◘ **Fig. 3.27** Inhomogeneous diaphragmatic nodular metastasis (*arrows*) adjacent to the right **a** and left **b** liver lobes

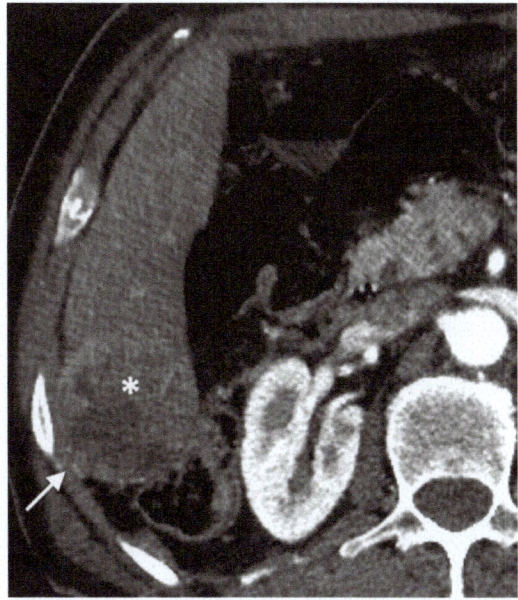

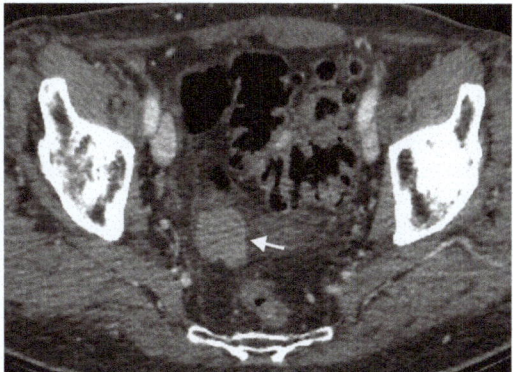

Fig. 3.30 Peritoneum dissemination of HCC (*arrow*)

References

1. Ferlay J, Soerjomataram II, Dikshit R et al (2014) Cancer incidence and mortality worldwide: sources, methods and major patterns in GLOBOCAN 2012. Int J Cancer 136:E359–E386
2. Njei B, Rotman Y, Ditah I, Lim JK (2015) Emerging trends in hepatocellular carcinoma incidence and mortality. Hepatology 61:191–199
3. European Association for the Study of the Liver; European Organisation for Research and Treatment of Cancer (2012) EASL-EORTC clinical practice guidelines: management of hepatocellular carcinoma. J Hepatol 56(4):908–943
4. Bucci L, Garuti F, Lenzi B, et al.; Italian Liver Cancer (ITA.LI.CA) Group (2016) The evolutionary scenario of hepatocellular carcinoma in Italy: an update. Liver Int. https://doi.org/10.1111/liv.13204. [Epub ahead of print]
5. Younossi ZM, Otgonsuren M, Henry L et al (2015) Association of nonalcoholic fatty liver disease (NAFLD) with hepatocellular carcinoma (HCC) in the United States from 2004 to 2009. Hepatology 62(6):1723–1730
6. Bruix J, Sherman M (2011) Management of hepatocellular carcinoma: an update. Hepatology 53:1020–1022
7. International Consensus Group for Hepatocellular Neoplasia (2009) Pathologic diagnosis of early hepatocellular carcinoma: a report of the International Consensus Group for Hepatocellular Neoplasia. Hepatology 49:658–664
8. Roncalli M, Terracciano L, Di Tommaso L, David E, Colombo M, Gruppo Italiano Patologi Apparato Digerente (GIPAD); Società Italiana di Anatomia Patologica e Citopatologia Diagnostica/International Academy of Pathology, Italian division (SIAPEC/IAP) (2011) Liver precancerous lesions and hepatocellular carcinoma: the histology report. Dig Liver Dis 43(suppl 4):S361–S372
9. Yamamoto T, Hirohashi K, Kaneda K et al (2001) Relationship of the microvascular type to the tumor size, arterialization and dedifferentiation of human hepatocellular carcinoma. Jpn J Cancer Res 92:1207–1213

Fig. 3.28 Large HCC in segment 6 (*asterisk*) with initial signs of capsular infiltration extending to the contiguous abdominal wall (*arrow*)

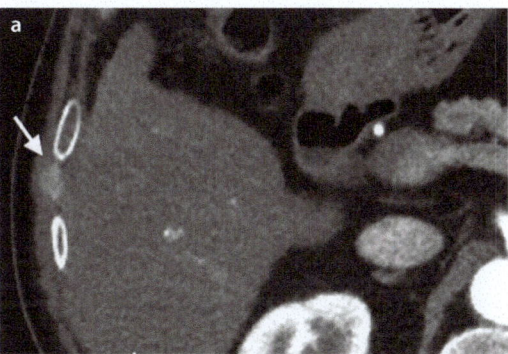

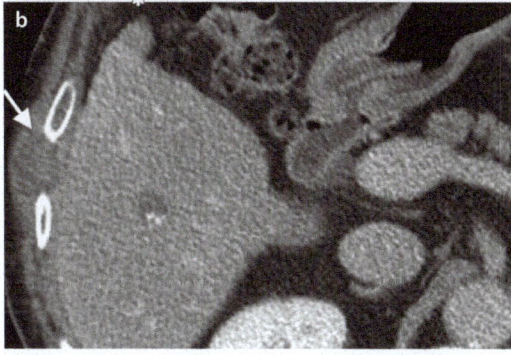

Fig. 3.29 Small metastasis of the abdominal wall (**a**, *arrow*) successfully treated by microwave ablation (**b**, *arrow*)

10. Park YN, Yang CP, Fernandez GJ, Cubukcu O, Thung SN, Theise ND (1998) Neoangiogenesis and sinusoidal "capillarization" in dysplastic nodules of the liver. Am J Surg Pathol 22:656–662

11. Choi JY, Lee JM, Sirlin CB (2014) CT and MR imaging diagnosis and staging of hepatocellular carcinoma: part I. Development, growth, and spread: key pathologic and imaging aspects. Radiology 272(3):635–654

12. Kudo M (2009) Multistep human hepatocarcinogenesis: correlation of imaging with pathology. J Gastroenterol 44(suppl 19):112–118

13. Roskams T, Kojiro M (2010) Pathology of early hepatocellular carcinoma: conventional and molecular diagnosis. Semin Liver Dis 30:17–25

14. Matsui O, Kobayashi S, Sanada J et al (2011) Hepatocellular nodules in liver cirrhosis: hemodynamic evaluation (angiography-assisted CT) with special reference to multi-step hepatocarcinogenesis. Abdom Imaging 36:264–272

15. Park HS, Lee JM, Kim SH et al (2009) Differentiation of well-differentiated hepatocellular carcinomas from other hepatocellular nodules in cirrhotic liver: value of SPIO-enhanced MR imaging at 3.0 tesla. J Magn Reson Imaging 29:328–335

16. Bartolozzi C, Crocetti L, Lencioni R, Cioni D, Della Pina C, Campani D (2007) Biliary and reticuloendothelial impairment in hepatocarcinogenesis: the diagnostic role of tissue-specific MR contrast media. Eur Radiol 17:2519–2530

17. Paradis V (2013) Histopathology of hepatocellular carcinoma. Recent Results Cancer Res 190:21–32

18. Adhoute X, Penaranda G, Raoul JL, Bourlière M (2016) Hepatocellular carcinoma scoring and staging systems. Do we need new tools? J Hepatol 64(6):1449–1450

19. Llovet JM, Brú C, Bruix J (1999) Prognosis of hepatocellular carcinoma: the BCLC staging classification. Semin Liver Dis 19(3):329–338

20. Bruix J, Reig M, Sherman M (2016) Evidence-based diagnosis, staging, and treatment of patients with hepatocellular carcinoma. Gastroenterology 150(4):835–853

21. Oken M, Creech R, Tormey D et al (1982) Toxicity and response criteria of the eastern cooperative oncology group. Am J Clin Oncol 5:649–655

22. Pugh RN, Murray-Lyon IM, Dawson JL, Pietroni MC, Williams R (1973) Transection of the oesophagus for bleeding oesophageal varices. Br J Surg 60:646–649

23. Livraghi T, Meloni F, Di Stasi M et al (2008) Sustained complete response and complications rates after radiofrequency ablation of very early hepatocellular carcinoma in cirrhosis: is resection still the treatment of choice? Hepatology 47:82–89

24. Cucchetti A, Piscaglia F, Cescon M et al (2013) Cost-effectiveness of hepatic resection versus percutaneous radiofrequency ablation for early hepatocellular carcinoma. J Hepatol 59:300–307

25. Roberts JP, Venook A, Kerlan R et al (2010) Hepatocellular carcinoma: ablate and wait versus rapid transplantation. Liver Transpl 16:925–929

26. Ferrer-Fàbrega J, Forner A, Liccioni A et al (2016) Prospective validation of "ab initio" liver transplantation in hepatocellular carcinoma upon detection of risk factors for recurrence after resection. Hepatology 63:839–849

27. Mazzaferro V, Regalia E, Doci R et al (1996) Liver transplantation for the treatment of small hepatocellular carcinomas in patients with cirrhosis. N Engl J Med 334(11):693–699

28. Yao FY, Ferrell L, Bass NM et al (2001) Liver transplantation for hepatocellular carcinoma: expansion of the tumor size limits does not adversely impact survival. Hepatology 33(6):1394–1403

29. Mazzaferro V, Llovet JM, Miceli R, et al.; Metroticket Investigator Study Group (2009) Predicting survival after liver transplantation in patients with hepatocellular carcinoma beyond the Milan criteria: a retrospective, exploratory analysis. Lancet Oncol 10(1):35–43

30. Clavien PA, Lesurtel M, Bossuyt PM, Gores GJ, Langer B, Perrier A, OLT for HCC Consensus Group (2012) Recommendations for liver transplantation for hepatocellular carcinoma: an international consensus conference report. Lancet Oncol 13(1):e11–e22

31. Majno P, Lencioni R, Mornex F, Girard N, Poon RT, Cherqui D (2011) Is the treatment of hepatocellular carcinoma on the waiting list necessary? Liver Transpl 17(Suppl 2):S98–108

32. Lu DS, Yu NC, Raman SS et al (2005) Radiofrequency ablation of hepatocellular carcinoma: treatment success as defined by histologic examination of the explanted liver. Radiology 234(3):954–960

33. Peng ZW, Zhang YJ, Chen MS et al (2013) Radiofrequency ablation with or without transcatheter arterial chemoembolization in the treatment of hepatocellular carcinoma: a prospective randomized trial. J Clin Oncol 31(4):426–432

34. Cha C, Fong Y, Jarnagin WR, Blumgart LH, DeMatteo RP (2003) Predictors and patterns of recurrence after resection of hepatocellular carcinoma. J Am Coll Surg 197:753–758

35. Lencioni R, Cioni D, Crocetti L et al (2005) Early-stage hepatocellular carcinoma in patients with cirrhosis: long-term results of percutaneous image-guided radiofrequency ablation. Radiology 234(3):961–967

36. Yang B, Zou J, Xia J et al (2011) Risk factors for recurrence of small hepatocellular carcinoma after long-term follow-up of percutaneous radiofrequency ablation. Eur J Radiol 79(2):196–200

37. Bruix J, Takayama T, Mazzaferro V et al.; STORM investigators (2015) Adjuvant sorafenib for hepatocellular carcinoma after resection or ablation (STORM): a phase 3, randomised, double-blind, placebo-controlled trial. Lancet Oncol 16(13):1344–1354

38. Llovet JM, Real MI, Montana X et al (2002) Arterial embolisation or chemoembolisation versus symptomatic treatment in patients with unresectable hepatocellular carcinoma: a randomised controlled trial. Lancet 359:1734–1739

39. Llovet JM, Bruix J (2003) Systematic review of randomized trials for unresectable hepatocellular carcinoma: chemoembolization improves survival. Hepatology 37:429–442

40. Lencioni R, de Baere T, Soulen MC, Rilling WS, Geschwind JF (2016) Lipiodol transarterial chemoembolization for hepatocellular carcinoma: a systematic review of efficacy and safety data. Hepatology 64(1):106–116

41. Burrel M, Reig M, Forner A et al (2012) Survival of patients with hepatocellular carcinoma treated by transarterial chemoembolisation (TACE) using drug eluting beads. Implications for clinical practice and trial design. J Hepatol 56:1330–1335

42. Malagari K, Pomoni M, Moschouris H et al (2012) Chemoembolization with doxorubicin-eluting beads for unresectable hepatocellular carcinoma: five-year survival analysis. Cardiovasc Intervent Radiol 35:1119–1128

43. Takayasu K, Arii S, Kudo M et al (2012) Superselective transarterial chemoembolization for hepatocellular carcinoma. Validation of treatment algorithm proposed by Japanese guidelines. J Hepatol 56:886–892

44. Lencioni R, Llovet JM, Han G et al (2016) Sorafenib or placebo plus TACE with doxorubicin-eluting beads for intermediate stage HCC: the SPACE trial. J Hepatol 64(5):1090–1098

45. Kudo M, Han G, Finn RS et al (2014) Brivanib as adjuvant therapy to transarterial chemoembolization in patients with hepatocellular carcinoma: a randomized phase III trial. Hepatology 60:1697–1707

46. Salem R, Lewandowski RJ, Kulik L et al (2011) Radioembolization results in longer time-to-progression and reduced toxicity compared with chemoembolization in patients with hepatocellular carcinoma. Gastroenterology 140(2):497–507

47. Moreno-Luna LE, Yang JD, Sanchez W et al (2013) Efficacy and safety of transarterial radioembolization versus chemoembolization in patients with hepatocellular carcinoma. Cardiovasc Intervent Radiol 36(3):714–723

48. Cucchetti A, Djulbegovic B, Tsalatsanis A et al (2015) When to perform hepatic resection for intermediate-stage hepatocellular carcinoma. Hepatology 61(3):905–914

49. Yao FY, Mehta N, Flemming J et al (2015) Downstaging of hepatocellular cancer before liver transplant: long-term outcome compared to tumors within Milan criteria. Hepatology 61(6):1968–1977

50. Bolondi L, Burroughs A, Dufour JF et al (2012) Heterogeneity of patients with intermediate (BCLC B) hepatocellular carcinoma: proposal for a subclassification to facilitate treatment decisions. Semin Liver Dis 32(4):348–359

51. Cheng AL, Kang YK, Chen Z et al (2009) Efficacy and safety of sorafenib in patients in the Asia-Pacific region with advanced hepatocellular carcinoma: a phase III randomised, double-blind, placebo-controlled trial. Lancet Oncol 10(1):25–34

52. Llovet JM, Ricci S, Mazzaferro V et al.; SHARP Investigators Study Group (2008) Sorafenib in advanced hepatocellular carcinoma. N Engl J Med 359(4): 378–390

53. Bruix J, Qin S, Merle P et al.; RESORCE Investigators (2017) Regorafenib for patients with hepatocellular carcinoma who progressed on sorafenib treatment (RESORCE): a randomised, double-blind, placebo-controlled, phase 3 trial. Lancet 389(10064):56–66

54. Mazzaferro V, Sposito C, Bhoori S et al (2013) Yttrium-90 radioembolization for intermediate-advanced hepatocellular carcinoma: a phase 2 study. Hepatology 57(5):1826–1837

55. Sangro B, Carpanese L, Cianni R et al.; European Network on Radioembolization with Yttrium-90 Resin Microspheres (ENRY) (2011) Survival after yttrium-90 resin microsphere radioembolization of hepatocellular carcinoma across Barcelona clinic liver cancer stages: a European evaluation. Hepatology 54(3):868–878

56. Gramenzi A, Golfieri R, Mosconi C et al.; BLOG (Bologna Liver Oncology Group) (2015) Yttrium-90 radioembolization vs sorafenib for intermediate-locally advanced hepatocellular carcinoma: a cohort study with propensity score analysis. Liver Int 35(3): 1036–1047

57. Kokudo T, Hasegawa K, Matsuyama Y et al.; Liver Cancer Study Group of Japan (2016) Survival benefit of liver resection for hepatocellular carcinoma associated with portal vein invasion. J Hepatol 65(5):938–943

58. Yau T, Tang VY, Yao TJ, Fan ST, Lo CM, Poon RT (2014) Development of Hong Kong liver cancer staging system with treatment stratification for patients with hepatocellular carcinoma. Gastroenterology 146(7): 1691–1700.e3

59. Kutami R, Nakashima Y, Nakashima O, Shiota K, Kojiro M (2000) Pathomorphologic study on the mechanism of fatty change in small hepatocellular carcinoma of humans. J Hepatol 33(2):282–289

60. ACR American College of Radiology. http://www.acr.org/Quality-Safety/Resources/LIRADS. Accessed 27 Oct 2016

61. Mitchell DG, Bruix J, Sherman M, Sirlin CB (2015) LI-RADS (Liver Imaging Reporting and Data System): summary, discussion, and consensus of the LI-RADS Management Working Group and future directions. Hepatology 61(3):1056–1065

62. Li M, Xin Y, Fu S et al (2016) Corona enhancement and mosaic architecture for prognosis and selection between of liver resection versus transcatheter arterial chemoembolization in single hepatocellular carcinomas >5 cm without extrahepatic metastases: an imaging-based retrospective study. Medicine (Baltimore) 95(2):e2458

63. Ishigami K, Yoshimitsu K, Nishihara Y et al (2009) Hepatocellular carcinoma with a pseudocapsule on gadolinium-enhanced MR images: correlation with histopathologic findings. Radiology 250(2):435–443

64. Iguchi T, Aishima S, Sanefuji K et al (2009) Both fibrous capsule formation and extracapsular penetration are powerful predictors of poor survival in human hepatocellular carcinoma: a histological assessment of 365 patients in Japan. Ann Surg Oncol 16(9):2539–2546

65. Nishie A, Yoshimitsu K, Asayama Y et al (2008) Radiologic detectability of minute portal venous invasion in hepatocellular carcinoma. AJR Am J Roentgenol 190(1):81–87

66. Kim H, Park MS, Choi JY et al (2009) Can microvessel invasion of hepatocellular carcinoma be predicted by pre-operative MRI? Eur Radiol 19(7):1744–1751

67. Sakon M, Nagano H, Nakamori S et al (2002) Intrahepatic recurrences of hepatocellular carcinoma after hepatectomy: analysis based on tumor hemodynamics. Arch Surg 137(1):94–99

68. Trevisani F, Cantarini MC, Wands JR, Bernardi M (2008) Recent advances in the natural history of hepatocellular carcinoma. Carcinogenesis 29(7):1299–1305

69. Wang J, Li Q, Sun Y et al (2009) Clinicopathologic features between multicentric occurrence and intrahepatic metastasis of multiple hepatocellular carcinomas related to HBV. Surg Oncol 18(1):25–30

70. Gouw AS, Balabaud C, Kusano H, Todo S, Ichida T, Kojiro M (2011) Markers for microvascular invasion in hepatocellular carcinoma: where do we stand? Liver Transpl 17(Suppl 2):S72–S80

71. Okamura S, Sumie S, Tonan T et al (2016) Diffusion-weighted magnetic resonance imaging predicts malignant potential in small hepatocellular carcinoma. Dig Liver Dis 48(8):945–952

72. Asman Y, Evenson AR, Even-Sapir E, Shibolet O (2015) [18F]fludeoxyglucose positron emission tomography and computed tomography as a prognostic tool before liver transplantation, resection, and loco-ablative therapies for hepatocellular carcinoma. Liver Transpl 21(5):572–580

73. Banerjee S, Wang DS, Kim HJ et al (2015) A computed tomography radiogenomic biomarker predicts microvascular invasion and clinical outcomes in hepatocellular carcinoma. Hepatology 62(3):792–800

74. Segal E, Sirlin CB, Ooi C et al (2007) Decoding global gene expression programs in liver cancer by noninvasive imaging. Nat Biotechnol 25(6):675–680

75. Nakashima Y, Nakashima O, Tanaka M, Okuda K, Nakashima M, Kojiro M (2003) Portal vein invasion and intrahepatic micrometastasis in small hepatocellular carcinoma by gross type. Hepatol Res 26(2):142–147

76. Reynolds AR, Furlan A, Fetzer DT et al (2015) Infiltrative hepatocellular carcinoma: what radiologists need to know. Radiographics 35(2):371–386

77. Engelbrecht M, Akin O, Dixit D, Schwartz L (2011) Bland and tumor thrombi in abdominal malignancies: magnetic resonance imaging assessment in a large oncologic patient population. Abdom Imaging 36(1):62–68

78. Ascenti G, Sofia C, Mazziotti S et al (2016) Dual-energy CT with iodine quantification in distinguishing between bland and neoplastic portal vein thrombosis in patients with hepatocellular carcinoma. Clin Radiol 71(9):938.e1-9

79. Catalano OA, Choy G, Zhu A, Hahn PF, Sahani DV (2010) Differentiation of malignant thrombus from bland thrombus of the portal vein in patients with hepatocellular carcinoma: application of diffusion-weighted MR imaging. Radiology 254(1):154–162

80. Sinn DH, Cho JY, Gwak GY et al (2015) Different survival of Barcelona clinic liver cancer stage C hepatocellular carcinoma patients by the extent of portal vein invasion and the type of extrahepatic spread. PLoS One 10(4):e0124434

81. Shi J, Lai EC, Li N et al (2011) A new classification for hepatocellular carcinoma with portal vein tumor thrombus. J Hepatobiliary Pancreat Sci 18(1):74–80

82. Yang T, Lin C, Zhai J et al (2012) Surgical resection for advanced hepatocellular carcinoma according to Barcelona Clinic Liver Cancer (BCLC) staging. J Cancer Res Clin Oncol 138(7):1121–1129

83. Prajapati HJ, Dhanasekaran R, El-Rayes BF et al (2013) Safety and efficacy of doxorubicin drug-eluting bead transarterial chemoembolization in patients with advanced hepatocellular carcinoma. J Vasc Interv Radiol 24(3):307–315

84. Kokudo T, Hasegawa K, Yamamoto S et al (2014) Surgical treatment of hepatocellular carcinoma associated with hepatic vein tumor thrombosis. J Hepatol 61(3):583–588

85. Zhang YF, Wei W, Guo ZX, Wang JH, Shi M, Guo RP (2015) Hepatic resection versus transcatheter arterial chemoembolization for the treatment of hepatocellular carcinoma with hepatic vein tumor thrombus. Jpn J Clin Oncol 45(9):837–843

86. Qiao W, Yu F, Wu L et al (2016) Surgical outcomes of hepatocellular carcinoma with biliary tumour thrombus: a systematic review. BMC Gastroenterol 16:11

87. Rammohan A, Sathyanesan J, Rajendran K et al (2015) Bile duct thrombi in hepatocellular carcinoma: is aggressive surgery worthwhile? HPB 17:508–513

88. Ueda M, Takeuchi T, Takayasu T et al (1994) Classification and surgical treatment of hepatocellular carcinoma (HCC) with bile duct thrombi. Hepato-Gastroenterology 41:349–354

89. Yoo JJ, Lee JH, Lee SH et al (2014) Comparison of the effects of transarterial chemoembolization for advanced hepatocellular carcinoma between patients with and without extrahepatic metastases. PLoS One 9(11):e113926

90. Natsuizaka M, Omura T, Akaike T et al (2005) Clinical features of hepatocellular carcinoma with extrahepatic metastases. J Gastroenterol Hepatol 20(11):1781–1787

91. Katyal S, Oliver JH 3rd, Peterson MS, Ferris JV, Carr BS, Baron RL (2000) Extrahepatic metastases of hepatocellular carcinoma. Radiology 216(3):698–703

92. Sneag DB, Krajewski K, Giardino A et al (2011) Extrahepatic spread of hepatocellular carcinoma: spectrum of imaging findings. AJR Am J Roentgenol 197(4):W658–W664

93. Uchino K, Tateishi R, Shiina S et al (2011) Hepatocellular carcinoma with extrahepatic metastasis: clinical features and prognostic factors. Cancer 117(19):4475–4483

94. Jung SM, Jang JW, You CR et al (2012) Role of intrahepatic tumor control in the prognosis of patients with hepatocellular carcinoma and extrahepatic metastases. J Gastroenterol Hepatol 27(4):684–689

95. Lee HS (2011) Management of patients with hepatocellular carcinoma and extrahepatic metastasis. Dig Dis 29(3):333–338

96. Kwon JB, Park K, Kim YD et al (2008) Clinical outcome after pulmonary metastasectomy from primary hepatocellular carcinoma: analysis of prognostic factors. World J Gastroenterol 14(37):5717–5722

97. Kitano K, Murayama T, Sakamoto M et al (2012) Outcome and survival analysis of pulmonary metastasectomy for hepatocellular carcinoma. Eur J Cardiothorac Surg 41(2):376–382

98. Hiraki T, Yamakado K, Ikeda O et al (2011) Percutaneous radiofrequency ablation for pulmonary metastases from hepatocellular carcinoma: results of a

multicenter study in Japan. J Vasc Interv Radiol 22(6):741–748

99. Kaczynski J, Hansson G, Wallerstedt S (1995) Metastases in cases with hepatocellular carcinoma in relation to clinicopathologic features of the tumor. An autopsy study from a low endemic area. Acta Oncol 34(1):43–48

100. Dodd GD 3rd, Baron RL, Oliver JH III, Federle MP, Baumgartel PB (1997) Enlarged abdominal lymph nodes in end-stage cirrhosis: CT-histopathologic correlation in 507 patients. Radiology 203(1):127–130

101. Kobayashi S, Takahashi S, Kato Y et al (2011) Surgical treatment of lymph node metastases from hepatocellular carcinoma. J Hepatobiliary Pancreat Sci 18(4):559–566

102. Mou Y, Zhao Q, Zhong L, Chen F, Jiang T (2016) Preliminary results of ultrasound-guided laser ablation for unresectable metastases to retroperitoneal and hepatic portal lymph nodes. World J Surg Oncol 14(1):165

103. Fukutomi M, Yokota M, Chuman H et al (2001) Increased incidence of bone metastases in hepatocellular carcinoma. Eur J Gastroenterol Hepatol 13(9):1083–1088

104. Seong J, Koom WS, Park HC (2005) Radiotherapy for painful bone metastases from hepatocellular carcinoma. Liver Int 25(2):261–265

105. Kashima M, Yamakado K, Takaki H et al (2010) Radiofrequency ablation for the treatment of bone metastases from hepatocellular carcinoma. AJR Am J Roentgenol 194(2):536–541

106. Ogura K, Miyake R, Shiina S et al (2012) Bone radiofrequency ablation combined with prophylactic internal fixation for metastatic bone tumor of the femur from hepatocellular carcinoma. Int J Clin Oncol 17(4):417–421

107. Hasegawa T, Yamakado K, Nakatsuka A et al (2015) Unresectable adrenal metastases: clinical outcomes of radiofrequency ablation. Radiology 277(2):584–593

108. Jung J, Yoon SM, Park HC et al (2016) Radiotherapy for adrenal metastasis from hepatocellular carcinoma: a multi-institutional retrospective study (KROG 13-05). PLoS One 11(3):e0152642

109. Park JS, Yoon DS, Kim KS et al (2007) What is the best treatment modality for adrenal metastasis from hepatocellular carcinoma? J Surg Oncol 96(1):32–36

110. Yamakado K, Anai H, Takaki H et al (2009) Adrenal metastasis from hepatocellular carcinoma: radiofrequency ablation combined with adrenal arterial chemoembolization in six patients. AJR Am J Roentgenol 192(6):W300–W305

Check for updates

Intrahepatic Cholangiocarcinoma

Maxime Ronot and Valérie Vilgrain

© Springer International Publishing AG 2018
D. Regge, G. Zamboni (eds.), *Hepatobiliary and Pancreatic Cancer*,
Cancer Dissemination Pathways, https://doi.org/10.1007/978-3-319-50296-0_4

4.1 Overview

4.1.1 Epidemiology

Intrahepatic cholangiocarcinoma (ICC) is a primary neoplasm that develops from epithelial cells of the intrahepatic bile ducts. It represents 10–15% of all primary liver cancers and is the second most common primary hepatic cancer after hepatocellular carcinoma [1]. It is associated with a very poor prognosis because most patients with ICC present with advanced disease, characterized by large multifocal tumors, vascular invasion, and in some cases extrahepatic spread.

4.1.2 Risk Factors

Cholangiocarcinogenesis is a multifactorial process. Several risks factors have been identified, but in the vast majority of cases, no risk factor is present. Long-established risk factors are hepatobiliary flukes (*Opisthorchis viverrini* and *Clonorchis*), primary sclerosing cholangitis (PSC), biliary inherited anomalies (choledochal cystic diseases, Caroli's disease), hepatolithiasis, and toxins. More recently, cirrhosis has been shown to be a risk factor.

4.1.3 Pathology

According to the Japanese Liver Cancer Group, different patterns of tumor growth can be described for ICC: mass-forming (exophytic), periductal (infiltrating), intraductal (polypoid), or mixed (mass-forming and periductal) pattern. Mass forming is the most frequent pattern in intrahepatic cholangiocarcinoma [2].

The pathological diagnosis of ICC is based on the WHO classification of biliary tract cancer. ICC is an adenocarcinoma or mucinous carcinoma with frequent marked fibrous stroma. Tumor spread is characterized by local intrahepatic metastases, vascular and perivascular invasion, lymphatic involvement, and perineural invasion, explaining both local and distant tumor spread patterns.

Local spread is driven by peritumoral intrahepatic metastases and vascular involvement. Intrahepatic local metastases are often referred to as "daughter" or "satellite" nodules and correspond to the growth of small tumors surrounding the main lesion. Local spread is different from that observed in hepatocellular carcinoma (HCC) and is more frequently macroscopic. Moreover, and unlike HCC, micro- and macrovascular spread are not endoluminal but perivascular and result in progressive vessel encasement.

Locoregional and more distant spread rely mostly on invasion and diffusion through the deep lymphatic system of the liver as well as on perineural invasion. The lymphatic system of the liver is divided into deep and superficial networks (▪ Fig. 4.1) [3]. The deep system follows the ramifications of the portal triads and hepatic veins, while the superficial system is in the connective tissue of convex and inferior surfaces of the liver. In the deep system, the periportal lymphatic tract is the most important, responsible for 80% of hepatic lymph drainage. Small lymphatics progressively merge into larger lymph vessels along the portal tract transporting lymph in the same direction as the bile, toward the hepatic hilum. The rich plexus of periportal tract lymphatics converges to form 12–15 lymph vessels that drain into the hepatic lymph nodes of the portal hilum. This explains the frequent hilar nodal extension of ICC. These hepatic lymph nodes are located along the hepatic vessels in the lesser omentum. The outgoing efferent lymphatic vessels from the perihilar lymph nodes reach the celiac lymph nodes, which drain into the cisterna chili (Pecquet cisterna) which is the dilated origin of the thoracic duct. The other part of the deep system contains lymphatics that follow the hepatic veins and merge into five to six large lymphatic vessels that pass through the diaphragm along with the inferior vena cava toward the posterior mediastinal lymph nodes [3]. This explains the possible presence of lung metastases as well as vascular invasion.

Perineural invasion is found at histopathology in up to 80% of patients. It is a known marker of highly aggressive disease and is associated with a poor prognosis [4–6]. The process of perineural invasion is different from metastases via the bloodstream or the lymphatic system, with distinctive histologic features, underlying cellular mechanisms, and molecular mediators [6].

4.1.4 Diagnosis

Imaging plays an important role in the diagnostic process as it allows assessment of locoregional and distant tumor spread. Imaging features of

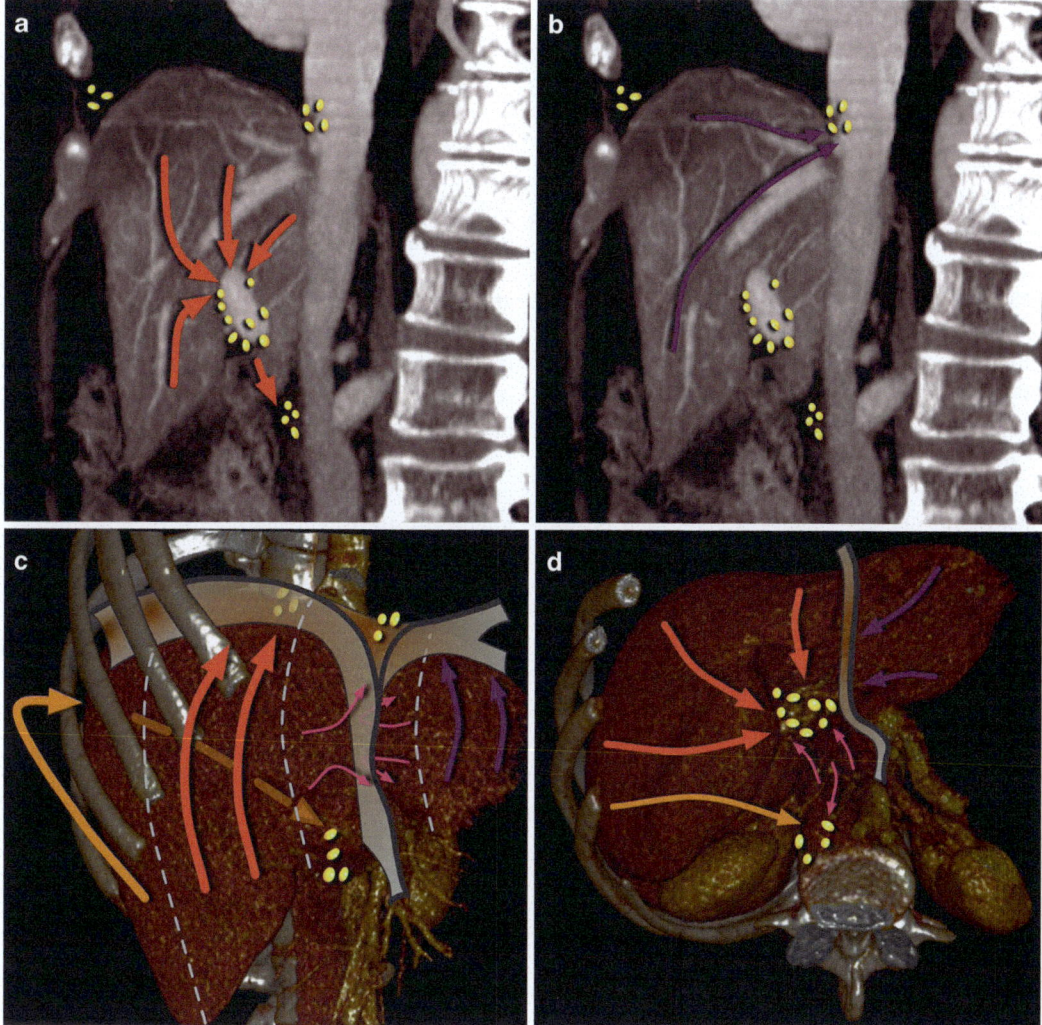

◘ Fig. 4.1 Schematic representation of the liver lymphatic system. **a** Deep lymphatic system of the liver—portal tract showing the course of the deep periportal lymphatic system (*red arrows*) to lymph nodes of the hepatic hilum and then to the celiac lymph nodes (*yellow dots*). **b** Deep lymphatic system of the liver—hepatic veins tract showing the course of the deep ascending lymphatic system (*purple arrows*) following hepatic veins to mediastinal lymph nodes (*yellow dots*). **c** Superficial lymphatic system of the liver. Right set (*orange arrow*): lymph vessels go by on the abdominal surface of the diaphragm to reach the celiac lymph nodes. Middle set (*red arrows*): through the inferior vena cava foramen to the mediastinal lymph nodes. Left set (*purple arrows*): through the esophageal hiatus to the superior gastric lymph nodes. Few central vessels (*pink arrows*) drain along the falciform ligament downward to the abdominal wall or upward to the parasternal lymph nodes. **d** Superficial lymphatic system of the liver—inferior surface. The majority of lymphatics (*red, purple and pink arrows*) converge toward the hepatic lymph nodes of *porta hepatis*. Few lymphatics of the posterior part of caudate and right lobes (orange and pink arrows) accompany the inferior vena cava through the diaphragm to mediastinal lymph nodes

ICC have been well described [1, 7]. The goal of imaging of ICC is threefold: (a) to characterize ICC by identifying suggestive imaging features, (b) to confirm the diagnosis with imaging-guided biopsy (c) to perform pre-therapeutic staging, and to assess surgical resectability. Several complementary imaging techniques are used to this purpose. Abdominal ultrasound (US) is often the first-line examination to identify tumor location and visualize upstream bile duct dilatation, when present. In experienced hands, US is a highly accurate diagnostic exam. However, a differential diagnosis and locoregional tumor extension cannot be determined with this technique. Multiphase

4

contrast-enhanced computed tomography (CT) and magnetic resonance imaging (MRI) are therefore performed to reach a positive and differential diagnosis of the lesion for tumor staging. Although CT accurately evaluates vascular encasement and provides whole-body imaging, MRI is the best technique to assess intrahepatic spread and biliary extension.

On unenhanced CT, ICC is usually seen as a hypoattenuating focal liver mass with irregular margins. Occasionally, calcifications may be seen. Multiphase contrast-enhanced CT acquisitions show peripheral rim enhancement on arterial phase images with progressive uptake on portal venous and delayed phases due to the presence of marked fibrous stroma [8]. CT may also frequently show biliary obstruction, capsular retraction, and/or ipsilateral parenchymal atrophy. On MR imaging, ICC is hypointense on T1-weighted and moderately hyperintense on T2-weighted images [9]. T2-weighted images may also show central hypointensity corresponding to areas of fibrosis. After extracellular contrast agent administration, dynamic images show peripheral enhancement on arterial phase images followed by progressive and concentric enhancement, somewhat similar to that observed with CT. If MR cholangiopancreatography is performed, it can help visualize the level of biliary obstruction, but the value of this technique is more limited than for hilar cholangiocarcinoma. Several enhancement patterns have been described on hepatospecific gadolinium chelate-enhanced MR imaging [10]. Most lesions (60%) show a thin peripheral rim with centripetal or progressive enhancement on portal venous phase images and marked hypointensity on hepatobiliary phase images (96%) [10].

The use of 18-fluorodeoxyglucose positron emission tomography (FDG-PET) to detect cholangiocarcinomas is a subject of debate. ICCs are usually considered to be FDG-avid lesions, and tumors as small as 1 cm can be detected with a reported sensitivity of 85–95%. However, FDG-PET is less accurate for identifying infiltrating tumors [11, 12]. Thus the clinical value of PET/CT for the diagnosis of ICC is limited when CT and/or MR imaging can identify typical features [13].

4.1.5 Staging

Optimal treatment of cholangiocarcinoma is based on complete tumor resection, which mainly depends on locoregional and distant tumor extension. The goal of surgery is to obtain complete tumor resection with safe margins (R0) while preserving a sufficient and functional future liver remnant, i.e., with good vascular in- and outflow and by restoring bile flow.

Unlike hilar cholangiocarcinoma, the literature on the staging of ICC is poor. However, several staging systems have been proposed, including two based on data from Japan [8, 9]. Okabayashi et al. [8] have proposed a staging system based on several independent factors associated with poor long-term survival, including the presence of vascular invasion, symptomatic disease, regional lymph node metastases, and multiple tumors (▶ Box 4.1). Yamasaki et al. [9] include tumor size (<2 cm or >2 cm), solitary vs. multiple tumors, the presence/absence of vascular or peritoneal invasion, distant metastases, and the presence/absence of regional lymph node metastases in their staging system (☐ Table 4.1). Recent studies have shown that prediction of the long-term prognosis was

---

Box 4.1   Proposed Staging System for Patients with Mass-forming Intrahepatic Cholangiocarcinoma According to Okabayashi et al. [17]

- T: Primary tumor
  - T1: Solitary tumor without vascular invasion
  - T2: Solitary tumor with vascular invasion
  - T3: Multiple tumors with or without vascular invasion
- N: Regional lymph nodes
  - N0: No regional lymph node metastases
  - N1: Regional lymph node metastases
- M: Distant metastasis
  - M0: No distant metastases
  - M1: Distant metastases
- Stage grouping
  - Stage I: T1 N0 M0
  - Stage II: T2 N0 M0
  - Stage IIIA: T3 N0 M0
  - Stage IIIB: Any T N1 M0
  - Stage IV: Any T any N M1

M metastasis status, *N* lymph node status, *T* tumor classification

◻ **Table 4.1** Proposed staging system for patients with mass-forming intrahepatic cholangiocarcinoma according to the Liver Cancer Study Group of Japan [14]

Criteria	
1. No. of tumors	Solitary
2. Size of largest tumor	2 cm
3. Venous or serosal invasion	
Tumor classification	
T1	All three criteria are fulfilled
T2	Only two of the three criteria are fulfilled
T3	Only one of the three criteria is fulfilled
T4	None of the three criteria are fulfilled
Stage	
I	T1N0M0
II	T2N0M0
III	T3N0M0
IVA	T4N0M0
	T1–T4N1M0
IVB	Any T any N M1

M metastasis status, *N* lymph node status, *T* tumor classification

Box 4.2 Proposed Staging System for Patients with Mass-forming Intrahepatic Cholangiocarcinoma According to Nathan et al. [18]

- T categories
  - T1: Solitary tumor, no vascular invasion
  - T2: Solitary tumor with vascular invasion
    - ≥ 2 tumors, ± vascular invasion
  - T3: Extrahepatic extension
- N categories
  - NX: Nearby (regional) lymph nodes cannot be assessed.
  - N0: No regional lymph node metastases
  - N1: Regional lymph node metastases
- M categories
  - M0: No distant metastases
  - M1: Distant metastases
- Stages
  - I T1, N0, M0
  - II T2, N0, M0 or T3, N0, M0
  - III Any T, N1, M0
  - IV Any T, any N, M1

Box 4.3 Proposed Staging System for Patients with Mass-forming Intrahepatic Cholangiocarcinoma According to the 7th edition of the AJCC [19]

- T categories
  - Tis: Cancer cells only in the mucosa (intramucosal carcinoma).
  - T1: Solitary tumor without vascular invasion
  - T2: Split into 2 groups:
    - T2a: Solitary tumor with vascular invasion
    - T2b: ≥2 tumors, ±vascular invasion
  - T3: Tumor perforating the visceral peritoneum or involving local extrahepatic structures by direct invasion
  - T4: Tumors with any periductal-infiltrating component
- N categories
  - N0: No regional lymph node metastases
  - N1: Regional lymph node metastases
- M categories
  - M0: No distant metastases
  - M1: Distant metastases
- Stages
  - 0 Tis, N0, M0
  - I T1, N0, M0
  - II T2, N0, M0
  - III T3, N0, M0
  - IVA T4, N0, M0 OR any T, N1, M0
  - IVB Any T, any N, M1

M metastasis status, *N* lymph node status, *T* tumor classification

poor with this staging system and have proposed a new one (▶ Box 4.2) [10]. In 2010 the 7th edition of the AJCC/UICCA staging manual was published, including a specific staging system for ICC (▶ Box 4.3) [11]. With the AJCC/UICCA system, tumor size is not considered a prognostic factor, while T-classification is based on the number of lesions, on the presence/absence of vascular invasion, intrahepatic metastasis, and invasion of adjacent structures. The AJCC/UICCA staging system also includes both "N" and "M" subclassifications. Regional lymph node metastases in the hilar, periduodenal, and peripancreatic nodes are considered N1 disease. This staging system has been independently validated [12] and endorsed by the European Association for the Study of the Liver (EASL) as the

4

preferred staging system for resected ICC (recommendation level B1) [1]. Nevertheless, EASL acknowledges that future studies should focus on stratifying nonsurgical patients for clinical studies using a clinical rather than a surgical staging process [1]. Recent reports suggest that the presence of metastatic lymph node or the analysis of lymph node ratio has better prognostic value than the AJCC 7th edition staging system [13]. These reports also stress that tumor size and biliary invasion should be reintroduced [14] (◘ Table 4.2), and that tumor growth types are essential [16].

◘ **Table 4.2** Proposed revised staging system for patients with mass-forming intrahepatic cholangiocarcinoma according to the Liver Cancer Study Group of Japan [15]

Criteria	
1. No. of tumors	Solitary
2. Size of largest tumor	2 cm
3. Vascular or major biliary invasion	vp0, va0, b0–b2
Tumor classification	
T1	All three criteria are fulfilled
T2	Only two of the three criteria are fulfilled
T3	Only one of the three criteria is fulfilled
T4	None of the three criteria are fulfilled
Stage	
I	T1N0M0
II	T2N0M0
III	T3N0M0
IVA	T4N0M0
	T1–T3N1M0
IVB	T4N1M0
	Any TN0, N1 M1

b0–b2 no biliary invasion or minor biliary invasion within second-order branch of the bile duct, *M* metastasis status, *N* lymph node status, *T* tumor classification, *va0* no arterial invasion, *vp0* no portal vein invasion

4.1.6 Treatment and Prognosis

Although surgery is the best-known treatment, only 20–40% of patients with ICC are eligible for potential curative resection at diagnosis [1]. Adjuvant chemotherapy and/or radiotherapy has failed to improve survival in most patients. The 5-year survival in patients following curative surgery is 30–35%, while the median overall survival is approximately 28 months [1]. ◘ Table 4.3 lists the main factors affecting survival in five different surgical series. The most important prognostic factors are age at diagnosis, tumor size (>2–3 cm), lymph node metastases, multiple tumors or intrahepatic metastases, vascular invasion [14, 16], and type of enhancement on contrast-enhanced CT [20]. Serosal invasion is not considered to be a prognostic factor in all studies [17, 21]. Multivariate analyses have shown that lymph node metastases, multiple tumors at presentation, and vascular invasion are the most important independent factors associated with a poor postoperative outcome [17, 18].

4.2 Patterns of Local Spread

4.2.1 Parenchymal Dissemination

According to Okabayashi et al., approximately one third of patients with a preoperative diagnosis of a solitary tumor have multiple satellite lesions in the resected specimen (◘ Fig. 4.2) [8]; when larger than 1 or 2 cm, approximately two thirds of satellite nodules are detected by imaging [20]. Historical studies have shown that CT and conventional MR imaging have similar performances for the detection of satellite lesions [17]. With both imaging modalities, nodules are appreciated because they enhance in parallel with the primary tumor. With the introduction of diffusion-weighted imaging (DWI) (◘ Fig. 4.3) and of hepatobiliary MR contrast agents, satellite nodules can be visualized better by MRI. Kang et al. reported additional daughter nodules (i.e., located around the main tumor) in 10% of the patients and intrahepatic metastases (i.e., distant from the main tumor) in 2%, using gadoxetic acid-enhanced MRI during the hepatobiliary phase [21]. CT or MR can be used to estimate the volume of the future liver remnant of potential surgical candidates. In patients with a healthy liver parenchyma,

□ Table 4.3 Recognized prognostic factors according to the main staging systems

	Okabayashi [17]	LCSGJ [14]	Nathan [18]	AJCC/UICC 7th [19]	LCSGJ revised [15]
Number of patients	60	136	598	598	419
Years	1981–1999	1990–1996	1988–2004	NM	2000–2005
Race	Japanese	Japanese	Western	Western	Japanese
Prognostic factors (worse survival)					
Tumor size	No	>2 cm	No	No	>2 cm
Tumor number	≥2	≥2	≥2	≥2	≥2
Vascular invasion	Yes	Yes	Yes	Yes	Yes
Peritoneal invasion	No	Yes	NM	Yes	Yes
Symptomatic tumor	Yes	NM	NM	NM	NM
Lymph node invasion	Yes	Yes	Yes	Yes	Yes
CEA preoperative	<5 ng/mL[a]	NM	NM	NM	NM
ALP preoperative	>300 IU/mL[a]	NM	NM	NM	NM
CA 19-9 preoperative	No	NM	NM	Yes	NM
R1 resection	No	No	NM	Yes	NM
PSC	No	NM	NM	Yes	NM

NM not mentioned in the original publication, *yes* significant prognostic factor, *no* no significant impact on survival, *ALP* alkaline phosphatase, *CA* carbohydrate antigen, *CEA* carcinoembryonic antigen, *LCSGJ* Liver Cancer Study Group of Japan, *PSC* primary sclerosing cholangitis
[a]Only significant prognostic factor in univariate analysis

25% of the total liver volume should be preserved to minimize morbidity from resection, whereas 40% of the total liver volume is required in patents with extensive fibrosis or cirrhosis. In patients with an insufficient future liver remnant, portal vein embolization (PVE) may be indicated to increase volume of remnant liver [18, 19]. Patients traditionally undergo sequential treatment with preoperative biliary drainage when necessary followed by PVE before resection.

4.2.2 Vascular Invasion

Assessment of vascular extension is important because it determines the therapeutic options and is predictive of oncological outcome. Unlike hepatocellular carcinoma, which spreads to the vascular lumen, progression of ICC results in vascular encasement. Imaging features suggestive for vascular involvement include close contact between the tumor and the vessel, vascular deformation, and stenosis or irregularities with nearly complete occlusion. Vascular encasement is present in approximately 50% of cases, and it involves the portal branches (□ Fig. 4.4) more often than the hepatic veins (□ Fig. 4.5) [20, 22]. The presence of segmental or lobar atrophy is strongly associated with ipsilateral portal vein encasement [23]. Anatomical variants (e.g., accessory right hepatic vein, low insertion of the right posterior portal vein, etc.) should be reported because it can change the treatment strategy.

Doppler ultrasound effectively identifies vascular invasion, encasement, or occlusion of both the portal veins and the hepatic arteries. In one study, preoperative US correctly identified 13/16 cases of liver tumors involving the hepatic vein yielding a sensitivity, specificity, and a PPV of 81%, 97%, and 87%, respectively [15]. In a second historical study,

4

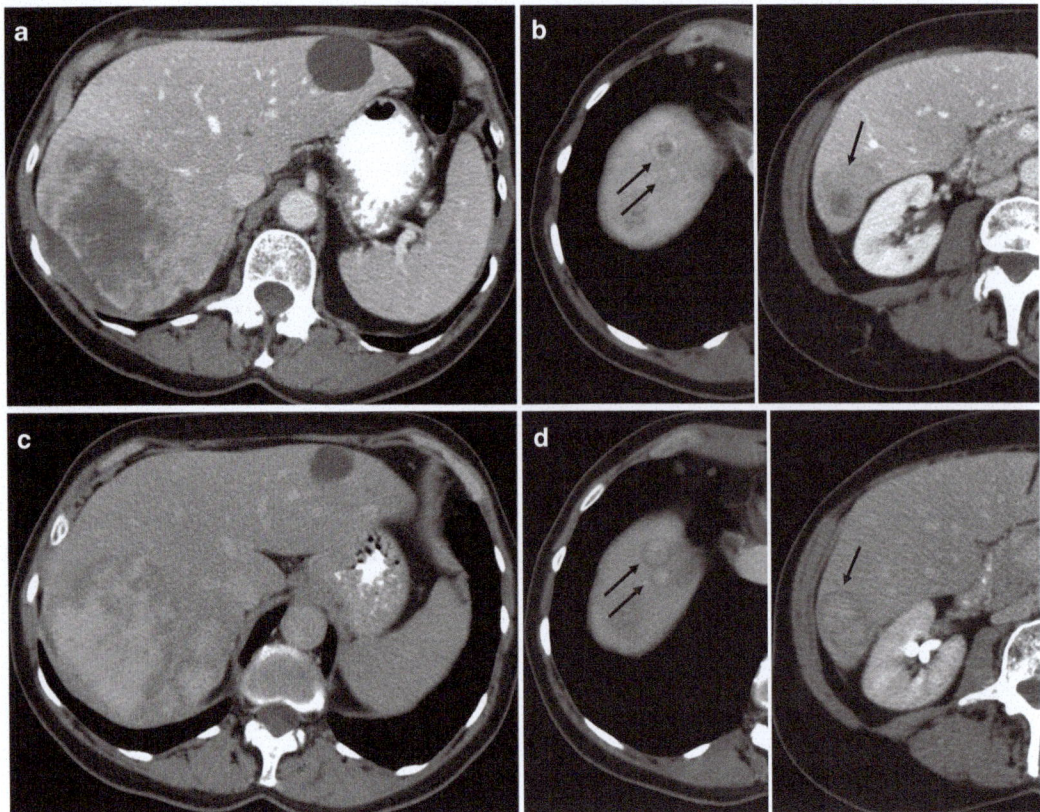

◘ **Fig. 4.2** Example of satellite nodules in a 63-year-old male with intrahepatic cholangiocarcinoma located in the right liver. Contrast-enhanced CT on portal venous **a**, **b** and delayed phase images **c**, **d** show a large heterogeneous mass with progressive enhancement (from **a** to **c**) and capsular retraction due to the presence of abundant fibrous stroma. Several smaller lesions (*arrows* in **b** and **d**) are depicted around the main tumor, with similar aspect. These lesions correspond to satellite nodules

preoperative US identified 38/41 patients (sensitivity = 93%) with portal vein involvement at surgery [24]. The above reported results were comparable to those of CT arterial portography. Nevertheless, in clinical practice the reference imaging modalities for vascular invasion are contrast-enhanced CT and MR imaging preferably with 3D and multiplanar reconstructions [25]. Although the two examinations are comparable, CT is considered more reliable in the assessment of vascular involvement due to its high spatial resolution.

4.3 Regional and Distal Spread

4.3.1 Lymph Node Involvement

It is important to accurately assess lymph nodal involvement as the presence of metastatic disease within the regional lymph nodes is a strong predictor of a poor long-term outcome following curative intent resection of intrahepatic cholangiocarcinoma [26]. Regional lymph nodes are divided into N1 nodes (hilum and around the common bile duct, periportal, peripancreatic, periduodenal) and N2 nodes (superior mesenteric and celiac). In published series, the overall accuracy of CT for detection of metastatic lymph nodes is 77%, and the most common error in preoperative imaging is underestimation of nodal involvement [20]. At CT neoplastic lymph nodes are round or enlarged and with a heterogeneous enhancement (◘ Figs. 4.6 and 4.7). Unfortunately, this pattern is uncommon in the early stage of lymph node involvement. Indeed, as previously reported, the size of the nodes is poorly correlated with tumor status since small nodes may be metastatic and large lymph nodes may be benign. For instance, Adachi et al. reported a 50% sensitivity for enlarged nodal size for the detection of tumor

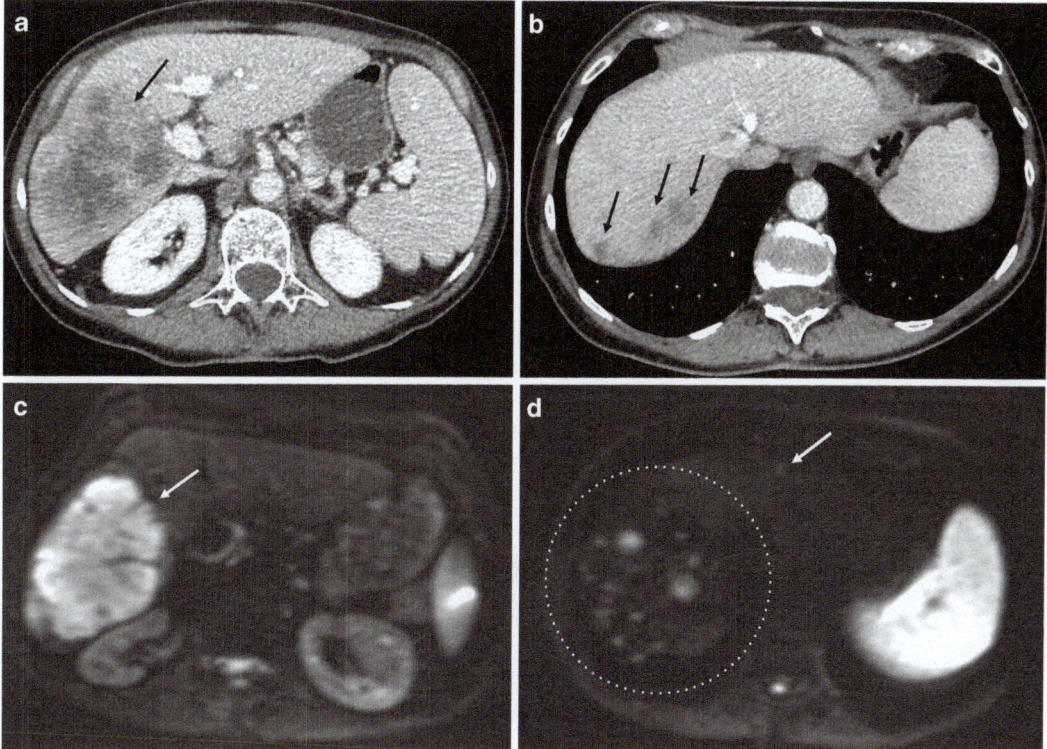

Fig. 4.3 Added value of diffusion-weighted images for the detection of satellite nodules in a 47-year-old male with intrahepatic cholangiocarcinoma located in the right liver. Contrast-enhanced CT on portal venous phase **a, b** shows a large heterogeneous mass in the right lobe (*arrow* in **a**) and several smaller lesions (*arrows* in **b**) located in the liver dome. On diffusion-weighted images **c, d** with high b values, the main tumor is more conspicuous (*arrow* in **c**). Images show significantly more satellite nodules in the liver dome (*dashed circle* in **d**) and a contralateral nodule (*arrow* in **d**)

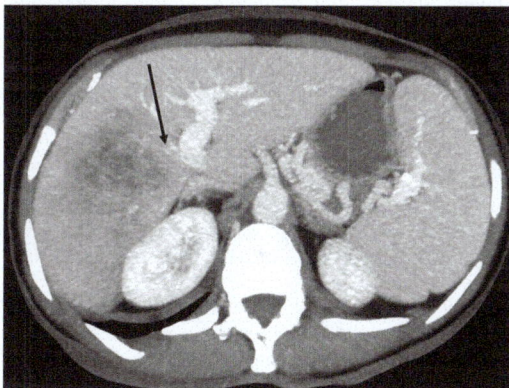

Fig. 4.4 Portal vein encasement in a 52-year-old male with intrahepatic cholangiocarcinoma of the right liver lobe. Contrast-enhanced CT with maximum intensity projection shows the heterogeneous mass in the right liver and the absence of right portal vein (*arrow*), due to the tumoral encasement. The main portal vein and the left branch were not involved

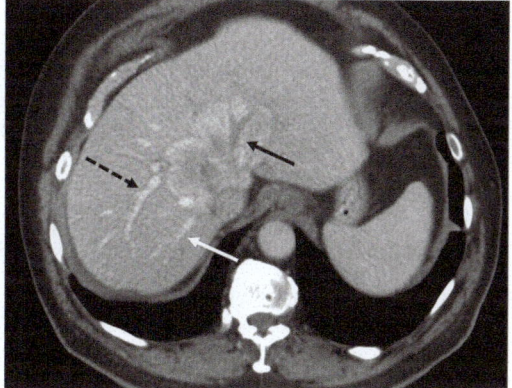

Fig. 4.5 Hepatic vein encasement in a 57-year old female with intrahepatic cholangiocarcinoma. Contrast-enhanced CT (portal venous phase) shows a heterogeneous mass located in the central part of the liver, in close contact with the inferior vena cava. The left hepatic vein is completely encased in the tumor and shows no contrast enhancement (*black arrow*). The right hepatic vein (*white arrow*) and the portal veins (*dashed arrow*) are not occluded

4

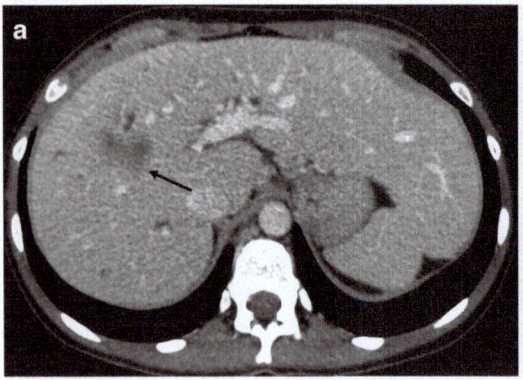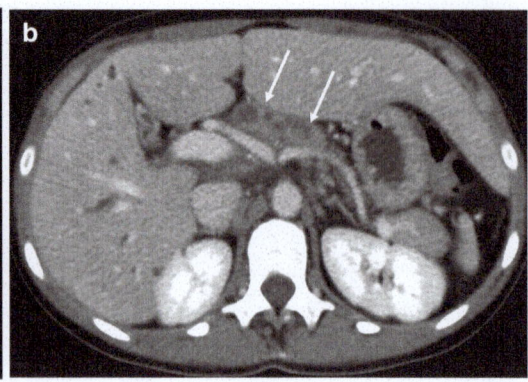

⬛ **Fig. 4.6** Metastatic lymph nodules in a 51-year-old female with intrahepatic cholangiocarcinoma. Contrast-enhanced CT (portal venous phase) shows a heterogeneous mass located in segment 8 (*arrow* in

a). Several enlarged and heterogeneous lymph nodes are depicted around along the liver vascular pedicle, around the hepatic and splenic arteries, and the celiac axis (*arrows* in **b**)

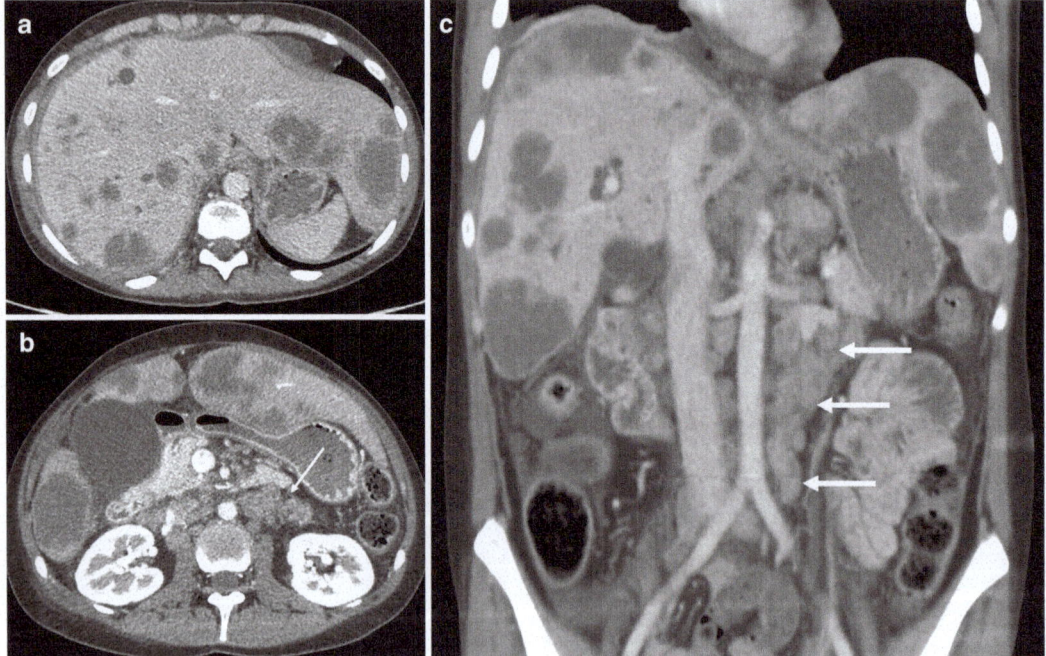

⬛ **Fig. 4.7** Retroperitoneal metastatic lymph nodules in a 68-year-old male with intrahepatic cholangiocarcinoma. Contrast-enhanced CT (portal venous phase) shows numerous bilobar hypodense tumors corresponding to

disseminated intrahepatic cholangiocarcinoma **a**. Multiple enlarged and heterogeneous lymph nodes are depicted in the retroperitoneum (*arrows* in **b** and **c**)

invasion [27]. Lymph nodes around the cardiac portion of the stomach and along the lesser gastric curvature should be examined in addition to nodes in the hepatoduodenal ligament in ICC of the left lobe [28].

Since at diffusion-weighted imaging, lymph nodes are hyperintense regardless of the tumoral status; there is no added value from this additional

sequence. Conversely, the use of hepatobiliary MR contrast agents could indirectly help in identifying nodal invasion. Indeed, Kang et al. have shown that the extent of relative enhancement of the main tumor on hepatobiliary phase images following Gd-EOB-DTPA administration was significantly higher in patients without than in those with lymph node metastases [21]. Finally, the diagnostic value of FDG-PET has been shown to be disappointing for the detection of regional lymph node metastases, even though its positive predictive value is higher than that of CT [29]. Thus, the contribution of preoperative imaging to determine malignant lymph nodes is low.

4.3.2 Perineural Invasion

The liver is innervated by both afferent and efferent autonomic nerves, which are associated with the portal vein, hepatic artery, and bile ducts within the liver hilum. The sympathetic innervation is postganglionic and originates in the celiac and superior mesenteric ganglia. The parasympathetic nerves branch off from the vagus nerve. The anterior plexus originates from the left portion of the celiac plexus and from the right abdominal branch of the vagus and forms a network of nerves surrounding the hepatic artery. The posterior plexus is derived from the right portion of the celiac plexus and is located around the portal vein with occasional innervations accompanying the hepatic vein (◘ Fig. 4.8a).

Perineural invasion is a common histological finding in biliary malignancies. It is a local diffusion mode for tumors, and it plays a critical role in prognosis [5]. Tumor perineural invasion is not correlated with patient's age or gender and with the presence of distant metastases (including liver or abdominal cavity or peritoneum metastases). However, it is highly correlated with tumor volume, location, depth of invasion, angiogenesis, and lymph node involvement [30]. The biliary system lies close to both the peripheral nervous plexus and the coeliac plexus, and this proximity may facilitate peripheral nerve invasion by biliary tumors. Since the biliary system is rich of autonomic nerves, perineural invasion may also be facilitated (◘ Fig. 4.8b) [31]. In the past it was thought that tumors invaded the nerves through the lymphatic pathway within the nerve or perineurium [30]. However, more recently it has been shown that not all patients presenting with perineural invasion have lymphatic metastasis [30]. By performing three-dimensional reconstruction of extrahepatic bile duct pathological specimens, Maxwell et al. [32] have shown that tumor perineural invasion is actually a type of local tumor growth pattern. Indeed, the perineural interspace invasion was the fifth dependent metastasis pathway to be discovered (aside from tumor direct invasion metastasis, implantation metastasis, lymphatic, and blood route metastasis). Farges et al. [26] have shown that in patients without lymph node invasion, a larger resection margin was associated with better survival, suggesting an important role of peritumoral perineural invasion.

Unfortunately there are few studies reporting imaging features of perineural invasion. However,

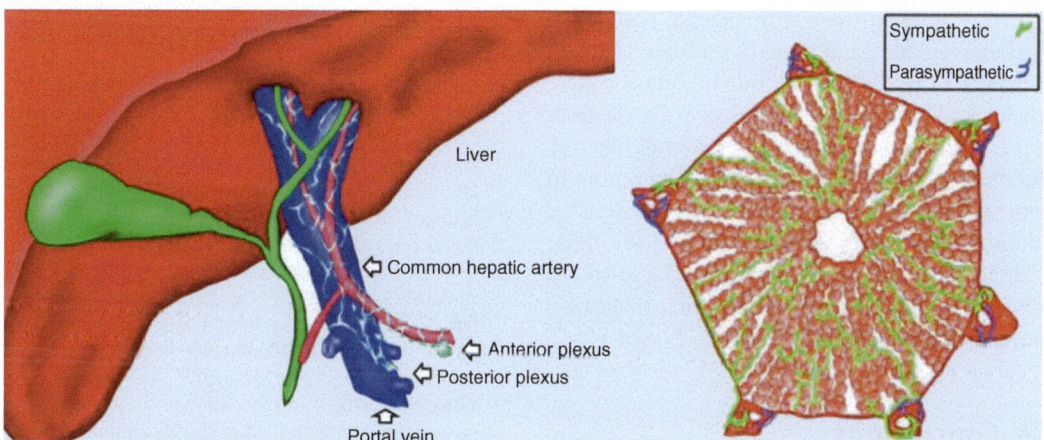

◘ **Fig. 4.8** **a** Gross anatomy of the hepatic nervous system. The anterior plexus forms around the common hepatic artery, and the posterior plexus forms around the portal vein. These plexuses follow these structures to enter the liver hilum with the accompanying portal structures and carry afferent and efferent fibers of both sympathetic and parasympathetic origin. **b** Anatomy of the intrinsic sympathetic and parasympathetic nerve fibers. Sympathetic and parasympathetic fibers surround the portal area, and sympathetic fibers course into liver sinusoids

Raghavan et al. demonstrated that soft-tissue infiltration along the celiac plexus on CT is a sign of perineural invasion [33]. This is surgically relevant because perineural invasion adjacent to the main tumor or within the gastrohepatic or the hepatoduodenal ligaments is potentially resectable with negative surgical margins. Conversely, celiac lymph node metastases or perineural invasion within the celiac plexus is generally a negative prognostic factor that contraindicates major hepatic resection with curative intent.

4.3.3 Distant Metastases

Extrahepatic and distant metastases of intrahepatic cholangiocarcinoma are rare at presentation, the most common sites being the lungs, peritoneum, and bones. At diagnosis, peritoneal carcinomatosis is rare, while it is more frequently observed as recurrence after resection. Whole-body CT and FDG-PET/CT are interesting complementary techniques to detect distant metastases. The main advantage of FDG-PET consists in the detection of otherwise unsuspected metastases, and its findings change the surgical management strategy in up to 30% of patients [34–36]. Thus, before surgical resection, PET/CT could be performed to help rule out occult metastatic disease.

Baheti et al. have shown that the features of the main tumor on CT affect the distribution pattern of distant metastases [37]. The authors identified three tumor types: type I, solitary dominant mass; type II, dominant mass with satellite nodules in the same segment; and type III, multiple scattered hepatic lesions. Solitary dominant masses were smaller and had the lowest incidence of metastases at presentation (26%) and the best overall survival. Pulmonary metastases were more common in patients with multiple scattered hepatic lesions, and bone metastases were less common in those with solitary dominant masses compared to the other groups. Finally, the time to first metastasis decreased from type I to type III [37].

4.4 Conclusions

Cholangiocarcinoma is the most common primary tumor of the bile ducts. Imaging plays an important role in the diagnosis of intrahepatic tumors which typically present as focal heterogeneous progressively enhancing mass, frequently associated with capsular retraction and upstream biliary dilatation. Definition of parenchymal, vascular, perineural, and nodal involvement as well as the identification of distant metastases with imaging is most important in order to select patients for curative resection. However, while imaging is accurate in detecting parenchymal invasion and vascular encasement, it has limitations in the evaluation of the extent of nodal and perineural invasion.

▪▪ Conflict of Interests

None of the authors have any conflict of interest or financial ties to disclose.

References

1. Bridgewater J, Galle PR, Khan SA, Llovet JM, Park JW, Patel T et al (2014) Guidelines for the diagnosis and management of intrahepatic cholangiocarcinoma. J Hepatol 60(6):1268–1289
2. The general rules for the clinical and pathological study of primary liver cancer. Liver cancer study group of Japan. Jpn J Surg 1989;19(1):98–129
3. Pupulim LF, Vilgrain V, Ronot M, Becker CD, Breguet R, Terraz S (2015) Hepatic lymphatics: anatomy and related diseases. Abdom Imaging 40(6):1997–2011
4. Mavros MN, Economopoulos KP, Alexiou VG, Pawlik TM (2014) Treatment and prognosis for patients with intrahepatic cholangiocarcinoma: systematic review and meta-analysis. JAMA Surg 149(6):565–574
5. Shirai K, Ebata T, Oda K, Nishio H, Nagasaka T, Nimura Y et al (2008) Perineural invasion is a prognostic factor in intrahepatic cholangiocarcinoma. World J Surg 32(11):2395–2402
6. Liebig C, Ayala G, Wilks JA, Berger DH, Albo D (2009) Perineural invasion in cancer: a review of the literature. Cancer 115(15):3379–3391
7. Kurzawinski TR, Deery A, Dooley JS, Dick R, Hobbs KE, Davidson BR (1993) A prospective study of biliary cytology in 100 patients with bile duct strictures. Hepatology 18(6):1399–1403
8. Okabayashi T, Yamamoto J, Kosuge T, Shimada K, Yamasaki S, Takayama T et al (2001) A new staging system for mass-forming intrahepatic cholangiocarcinoma: analysis of preoperative and postoperative variables. Cancer 92(9):2374–2383
9. Yamasaki S (2003) Intrahepatic cholangiocarcinoma: macroscopic type and stage classification. J Hepato-Biliary-Pancreat Surg 10(4):288–291
10. Nathan H, Aloia TA, Vauthey JN, Abdalla EK, Zhu AX, Schulick RD et al (2009) A proposed staging system for intrahepatic cholangiocarcinoma. Ann Surg Oncol 16(1):14–22

11. Edge SB, Compton CC (2010) The American Joint Committee on Cancer: the 7th edition of the AJCC cancer staging manual and the future of TNM. Ann Surg Oncol 17(6):1471–1474

12. Farges O, Fuks D, Le Treut YP, Azoulay D, Laurent A, Bachellier P et al (2011) AJCC 7th edition of TNM staging accurately discriminates outcomes of patients with resectable intrahepatic cholangiocarcinoma: by the AFC-IHCC-2009 Study Group. Cancer 117(10): 2170–2177

13. Kim Y, Spolverato G, Amini N, Margonis GA, Gupta R, Ejaz A et al (2015) Surgical management of intrahepatic cholangiocarcinoma: defining an optimal prognostic lymph node stratification schema. Ann Surg Oncol 22(8):2772–2778

14. Sakamoto Y, Kokudo N, Matsuyama Y, Sakamoto M, Izumi N, Kadoya M et al (2016) Proposal of a new staging system for intrahepatic cholangiocarcinoma: analysis of surgical patients from a nationwide survey of the Liver Cancer Study Group of Japan. Cancer 122(1):61–70

15. Hann LE, Schwartz LH, Panicek DM, Bach AM, Fong Y, Blumgart LH (1998) Tumor involvement in hepatic veins: comparison of MR imaging and US for preoperative assessment. Radiology 206(3):651–656

16. Hwang S, Lee YJ, Song GW, Park KM, Kim KH, Ahn CS et al (2015) Prognostic impact of tumor growth type on 7th AJCC staging system for intrahepatic cholangiocarcinoma: a single-center experience of 659 cases. J Gastrointest Surg 19(7):1291–1304

17. Zhang Y, Uchida M, Abe T, Nishimura H, Hayabuchi N, Nakashima Y (1999) Intrahepatic peripheral cholangiocarcinoma: comparison of dynamic CT and dynamic MRI. J Comput Assist Tomogr 23(5):670–677

18. Madoff DC, Hicks ME, Abdalla EK, Morris JS, Vauthey JN (2003) Portal vein embolization with polyvinyl alcohol particles and coils in preparation for major liver resection for hepatobiliary malignancy: safety and effectiveness—study in 26 patients. Radiology 227(1):251–260

19. Kubota K, Makuuchi M, Kusaka K, Kobayashi T, Miki K, Hasegawa K et al (1997) Measurement of liver volume and hepatic functional reserve as a guide to decision-making in resectional surgery for hepatic tumors. Hepatology 26(5):1176–1181

20. Vilgrain V (2008) Staging cholangiocarcinoma by imaging studies. HPB (Oxford) 10(2):106–109

21. Kang Y, Lee JM, Kim SH, Han JK, Choi BI (2012) Intrahepatic mass-forming cholangiocarcinoma: enhancement patterns on gadoxetic acid-enhanced MR images. Radiology 264(3):751–760

22. Vilgrain V, Van Beers BE, Flejou JF, Belghiti J, Delos M, Gautier AL et al (1997) Intrahepatic cholangiocarcinoma: MRI and pathologic correlation in 14 patients. J Comput Assist Tomogr 21(1):59–65

23. Feydy A, Vilgrain V, Denys A, Sibert A, Belghiti J, Vullierme MP et al (1999) Helical CT assessment in hilar cholangiocarcinoma: correlation with surgical and pathologic findings. AJR Am J Roentgenol 172(1):73–77

24. Bach AM, Hann LE, Brown KT, Getrajdman GI, Herman SK, Fong Y et al (1996) Portal vein evaluation with US:

comparison to angiography combined with CT arterial portography. Radiology 201(1):149–154

25. Uchida M, Ishibashi M, Tomita N, Shinagawa M, Hayabuchi N, Okuda K (2005) Hilar and suprapancreatic cholangiocarcinoma: value of 3D angiography and multiphase fusion images using MDCT. AJR Am J Roentgenol 184(5):1572–1577

26. Farges O, Fuks D, Boleslawski E, Le Treut YP, Castaing D, Laurent A et al (2011) Influence of surgical margins on outcome in patients with intrahepatic cholangiocarcinoma: a multicenter study by the AFC-IHCC-2009 study group. Ann Surg 254(5):824–829, discussion 30

27. Adachi T, Eguchi S, Beppu T, Ueno S, Shiraishi M, Okuda K et al (2015) Prognostic impact of preoperative lymph node enlargement in intrahepatic cholangiocarcinoma: a multi-institutional study by the Kyushu Study Group of Liver Surgery. Ann Surg Oncol 22(7):2269–2278

28. Okami J, Dono K, Sakon M, Tsujie M, Hayashi N, Fujiwara Y et al (2003) Patterns of regional lymph node involvement in intrahepatic cholangiocarcinoma of the left lobe. J Gastrointest Surg 7(7):850–856

29. Lee SW, Kim HJ, Park JH, Park DI, Cho YK, Sohn CI et al (2010) Clinical usefulness of 18F-FDG PET-CT for patients with gallbladder cancer and cholangiocarcinoma. J Gastroenterol 45(5):560–566

30. Shen FZ, Zhang BY, Feng YJ, Jia ZX, An B, Liu CC et al (2010) Current research in perineural invasion of cholangiocarcinoma. J Exp Clin Cancer Res 29:24

31. Murakawa K, Tada M, Takada M, Tamoto E, Shindoh G, Teramoto K et al (2004) Prediction of lymph node metastasis and perineural invasion of biliary tract cancer by selected features from cDNA array data. J Surg Res 122(2):184–194

32. Maxwell P, Hamilton PW, Sloan JM (1996) Three-dimensional reconstruction of perineural invasion in carcinoma of the extrahepatic bile ducts. J Pathol 180(2):142–145

33. Raghavan K, Jeffrey RB, Patel BN, DiMaio MA, Willmann JK, Olcott EW (2015) MDCT diagnosis of perineural invasion involving the celiac plexus in intrahepatic cholangiocarcinoma: preliminary observations and clinical implications. AJR Am J Roentgenol 205(6):W578–W584

34. Anderson CD, Rice MH, Pinson CW, Chapman WC, Chari RS, Delbeke D (2004) Fluorodeoxyglucose PET imaging in the evaluation of gallbladder carcinoma and cholangiocarcinoma. J Gastrointest Surg 8(1):90–97

35. Corvera CU, Blumgart LH, Akhurst T, DeMatteo RP, D'Angelica M, Fong Y et al (2008) 18F-fluorodeoxyglucose positron emission tomography influences management decisions in patients with biliary cancer. J Am Coll Surg 206(1):57–65

36. Kim YJ, Yun M, Lee WJ, Kim KS, Lee JD (2003) Usefulness of 18F-FDG PET in intrahepatic cholangiocarcinoma. Eur J Nucl Med Mol Imaging 30(11):1467–1472

37. Baheti AD, Tirumani SH, Shinagare AB, Rosenthal MH, Hornick JL, Ramaiya NH et al (2014) Correlation of CT patterns of primary intrahepatic cholangiocarcinoma at the time of presentation with the metastatic spread and clinical outcomes: retrospective study of 92 patients. Abdom Imaging 39(6):1193–1201

Bile Duct and Gallbladder Tumors

Stefano Cirillo, Alessandro Ferrero, Teresa Gallo,
Nadia Russolillo, and Stefano Cavanna

© Springer International Publishing AG 2018
D. Regge, G. Zamboni (eds.), *Hepatobiliary and Pancreatic Cancer,*
Cancer Dissemination Pathways, https://doi.org/10.1007/978-3-319-50296-0_5

5.1 Overview

5.1.1 Epidemiology

Bile duct carcinoma is rare, accounting for <2% of all tumors [1–3]. Its prevalence varies according to geographic region, with the highest rates reported in Southeast Asia, partly due to endemic liver parasitic infections. According to the American Cancer Society, about 2–3000 people in the USA develop cholangiocarcinoma each year [2]. Recent reports have shown that incidence and mortality are increasing, especially in Western Europe and the USA, but this data may be in part attributed to misclassification of intra- and extrahepatic cholangiocarcinomas [3]. The average age of presentation is 60–70 years, with a slightly male predilection (54%) [2, 4].

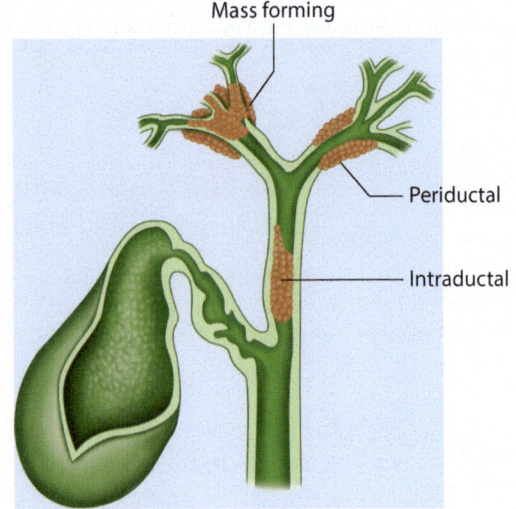

● **Fig. 5.1**   Different growth types of hilar cholangiocarcinoma according to Liver Cancer Study Groups, Japan

5.1.2 Risk Factors

Most cholangiocarcinomas develop without a specific etiology, but a strong correlation between tumor development and any condition leading to a state of chronic irritation or inflammation and cholestasis in the biliary tree has been observed [5]. Numerous risk factors have been identified including [5] primary sclerosing cholangitis, recurrent pyogenic cholangitis, cholelithiasis, hepatobiliary flukes (*Opisthorchis viverrini*, *Clonorchis sinensis*), Caroli's disease/choledochal cysts, congenital hepatic fibrosis, toxins (thorotrast, polyvinyl chloride, heavy alcohol use), viral infections (HIV, HBV, HCV, EBV), cirrhosis, and other abnormalities of the biliary duct (especially those with pancreatic juice reflux in the bile duct).

5.1.3 Pathology

More than 95% of biliary tract neoplasms are cholangiocarcinomas, a malignant tumor arising from the biliary tract epithelium, while other types of bile duct tumors, i.e., sarcomas, small cell cancers, etc., are very rare. The Liver Cancer Study Group of Japan classifies bile duct cholangiocarcinoma based on the type of growth considering the following three major classes (● Fig. 5.1): mass-forming or nodular type, periductal-infiltrating or sclerosing type, and intraductal-growing or papillary type. This classification directly correlates

with the overall survival of patients, the longest survival being that of the papillary type followed by the mass-forming type [4].

Cholangiocarcinoma may arise from any part of the biliary tree (● Fig. 5.2). The most common site of origin is the hepatic hilum followed by the distal bile duct and the intrahepatic bile ducts. The first two locations together are defined as extrahepatic bile duct cancers. Hilar cholangiocarcinoma, or Klatskin's tumor, is by far the most common site of bile duct cancer accounting for approximately two thirds of cases. Cholangiocarcinoma develops through multistep carcinogenesis, and two types of precursor lesions have been identified: a flat intraepithelial biliary neoplasia or Bilin (discernible only at a microscopic level) and an intraductal papillary lesion or IPNB (previously named papillomatosis) [6]. Both these lesions arise in large hilar and extrahepatic bile ducts and are only rarely present in the septal or interlobular bile ducts.

Cholangiocarcinomas may also originate from the fundus (60%), body (30%), or neck (10%) of the gallbladder [6]. The latter, likewise hilar cholangiocarcinoma, has two types of precursor lesions: flat lesions with either low-grade dysplasia or high-grade dysplasia and mass-forming lesions (adenomas). Most of gallbladder carcinomas arise from flat dysplasia, while mass-forming precursor lesions are found only in few cases [7–10].

■ **Fig. 5.2** Classification of cholangiocarcinoma according to tumor location

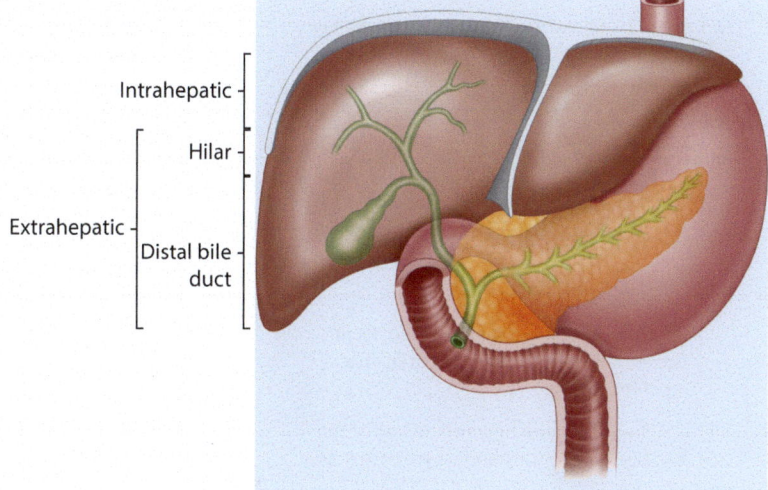

Intrahepatic

Hilar

Extrahepatic

Distal bile duct

5.1.4 Staging

To date, there is no optimal pathologic staging system for bile duct cholangiocarcinoma that provides both good prognostic capabilities and aids in surgical planning and patient selection. The most widespread staging system for cholangiocarcinomas is the 2010 American Joint Committee on Cancer (AJCC) TNM system. The system includes four separate staging systems, based on primary tumor site (■ Tables 5.1 and 5.2) [11]. A new staging system for hilar carcinoma based on published prognostic factors and resectability criteria has been recently proposed, but it still needs to be validated in large patient series (■ Table 5.3) [12].

Biliary involvement of hilar carcinomas can be classified according to the Bismuth-Corlette classification (■ Fig. 5.3). This classification is not a staging system but an anatomic description originally developed to assess resectability of hilar cholangiocarcinomas [13, 14].

■ **Table 5.1** Gallbladder cancer staging according to AJCC (7th edn, 2010)

Gallbladder cancer staging	
Primary tumor (T)	
TX	Primary tumor cannot be assessed
T0	No evidence of primary tumor
Tis	Carcinoma in situ
T1	Tumor invades lamina propria or muscular layer

■ **Table 5.1** (continued)

Gallbladder cancer staging	
T1a	Tumor invades lamina propria
T1b	Tumor invades muscular layer
T2	Tumor invades perimuscular connective tissue, no extension beyond the serosa or into the liver
T3	Tumor perforates the serosa (visceral peritoneum) and/or directly invades the liver and/or one other adjacent organ or structure, such as the stomach, duodenum, colon, pancreas, omentum, or extrahepatic bile ducts
T4	Tumor invades main portal vein or hepatic artery or invades 2 or more extrahepatic organs or structures
Regional lymph nodes (N)	
NX	Regional lymph nodes cannot be assessed
N0	No regional lymph node metastasis
N1	Metastases to nodes along the cystic duct, common bile duct, hepatic artery, and/or portal vein
N2	Metastases to periaortic, pericaval, superior mesenteric artery, and/or celiac artery lymph nodes
Distant metastasis (M)	
M0	No distant metastasis
M1	Distant metastasis

◻ **Table 5.2**   Hilar cholangiocarcinoma staging according to AJCC (7th edn, 2010)

	Hilar cholangiocarcinoma staging
Primary tumor (T)	
TX	Primary tumor cannot be assessed
T0	No evidence of primary tumor
Tis	Carcinoma in situ
T1	Tumor confined to the bile duct, with extension up to the muscle layer or fibrous tissue
T2a	Tumor invades beyond the wall of the bile duct to surrounding adipose tissue
T2b	Tumor invades adjacent hepatic parenchyma
T3	Tumor invades unilateral branches of the portal vein or hepatic artery
T4	Tumor invades main portal vein or its branches bilaterally, the common hepatic artery, the second-order biliary radicals bilaterally, or the second-order biliary radicals unilaterally, with contralateral portal vein or hepatic artery involvement
Regional lymph nodes (N)	
NX	Regional lymph nodes cannot be assessed
N0	No regional lymph node metastasis
N1	Regional lymph node metastasis (including nodes along the cystic duct, common bile duct, hepatic artery, and portal vein)
N2	Metastasis to periaortic, pericaval, superior mesenteric artery, and/or celiac artery lymph nodes
Distant metastasis (M)	
M0	No distant metastasis
M1	Distant metastasis

◻ **Table 5.3**   Hilar cholangiocarcinoma staging system proposed by Deoliveira et al

	Side/location	Description
Bile duct (B) (based on Bismuth classification)		
B1		Common bile duct
B2		Hepatic duct confluence
B3	R	Right hepatic duct
B3	L	Left hepatic duct
B4		Right and left hepatic duct
Tumor size (T)		
T1		<1 cm
T2		1–<3 cm
T3		≥3 cm
Tumor form (F)		
Sclerosing		Sclerosing (or periductal)
Mass		Mass forming (or nodular)
Mixed		Sclerosing and mass forming
Polypoid		Polypoid (or intraductal)
Involvement (>180°) of the portal vein (PV)		
PV0		No portal involvement
PV1		Main portal vein
PV2		Portal vein bifurcation
PV3	R	Right portal vein
PV3	L	Left portal vein
PV4		Right and left portal vein
Involvement (>180°) of the hepatic artery (HA)		
HA0		No arterial involvement
HA1		Proper hepatic artery
HA2		Hepatic artery bifurcation
HA3	R	Right hepatic artery
HA3	L	Left hepatic artery
HA4		Right and left hepatic artery
Liver remnant volume (V)		
V0		No information on volume needed (liver resection not foreseen)

5.1.5 Diagnosis

5.1.5.1 Bile Duct Carcinoma

Accurate assessment of both local and distant dissemination is mandatory for treatment planning. Bile duct carcinoma may spread both vertically and horizontally (◻ Fig. 5.4). *Vertical spread* occurs when

▣ Table 5.3 (continued)		
	Side/ location	Description
V (%)	Indicate segments	% total volume of a putative remnant liver after resection
Lymph nodes (N) (based on Japanese Society of Biliary Surgery)		
N0		No lymph nodes involvement
N1		Hilar and/or hepatic artery lymph nodes involvement
N2		Periaortic lymph nodes involvement
Metastases (M) (based on TNM classification (11))		
M0		No distant metastases
M1		Distant metastases, including liver and peritoneal metastases

tumor disseminates to the adjacent tissues, more commonly to the liver parenchyma, portal venous system, hepatic artery, and regional lymph nodes. *Horizontal spread* occurs when tumor progresses along the bile duct long axis. Progression along the bile ducts in one of the decisive factors determining resectability and in case surgery is decided upon the extent of liver resection. Involvement beyond the second branch on both sides is a criterion of non-resectability [14, 15]. Intraepithelial spread of bile duct carcinoma has been found in over 10% of patients, but it is difficult to diagnose because the cancer cells replace the normal epithelium of the bile ducts without any perceptible thickening of ducts walls (a thickening less than 1 mm is considered impossible to prove with imaging techniques) [16, 17].

Computed tomography (CT) is the best imaging modality to evaluate the spread of bile duct carcinomas into the surrounding tissues and the relationship between tumor and the vascular structures within the hepatic pedicle. CT should be performed using a multiphasic technique, which should include a delayed phase, starting 150–180 s from intravenous iodine injection. Bile duct cancer may show a

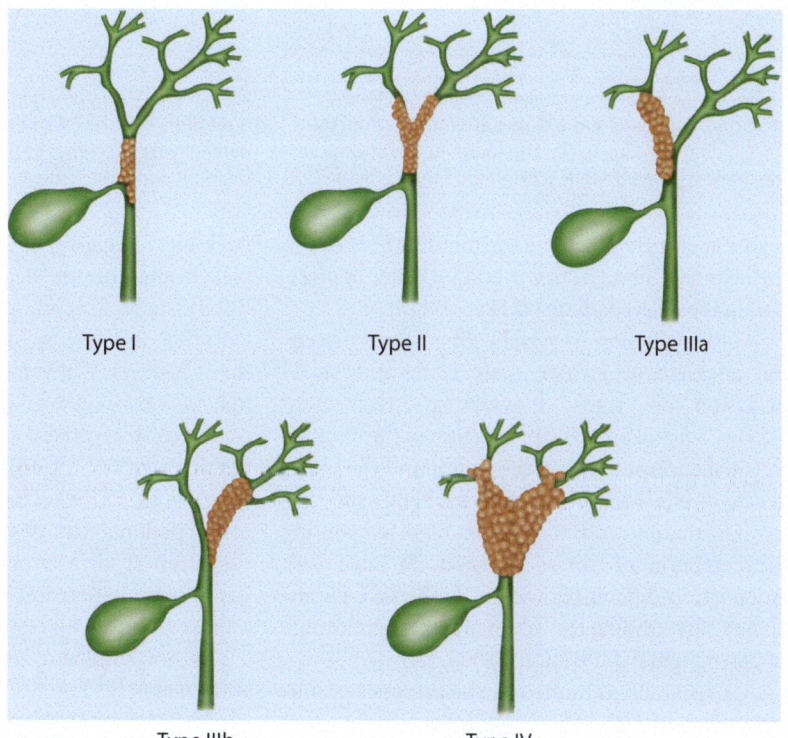

▣ **Fig. 5.3** Bismuth-Corlette classification of hilar cholangiocarcinoma. Type I: tumor limited to the common hepatic duct, below the level of the confluence of the right and left hepatic ducts. Type II: tumor involves the right and left hepatic ducts. Type IIIa: tumor extends to the right hepatic duct. Type IIIb: tumor extends to the left hepatic duct. Type IV: tumor extends to the bifurcations of both right and left hepatic ducts or multifocal involvement

Type I   Type II   Type IIIa

Type IIIb   Type IV

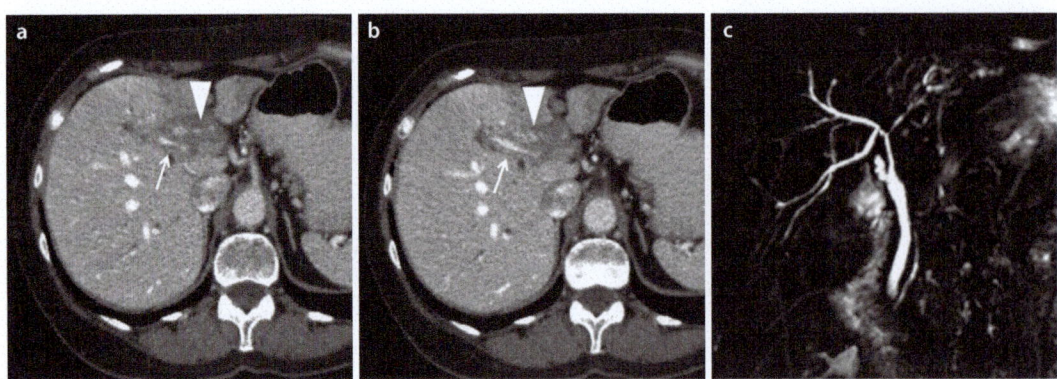

Fig. 5.4   **a, b** CT shows infiltration of both the left portal vein (*white arrow*) and artery (*arrow head*, vertical spread); **c** MRCP shows left bile duct involvement (horizontal spread)

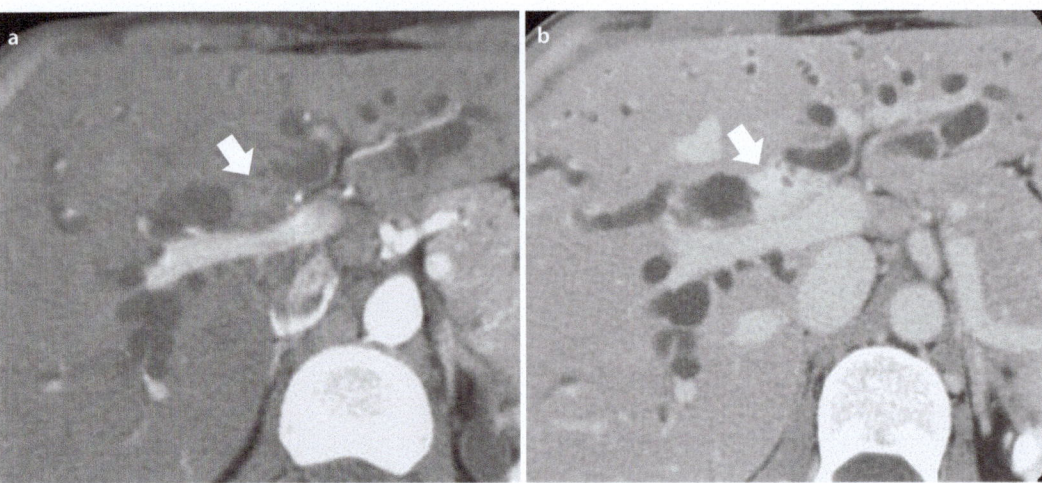

Fig. 5.5   CT scan shows hilar cholangiocarcinoma (*white arrows*). Tumor has a higher attenuation than the surrounding liver due to the abundant fibrous stroma in the delayed phase **b**, while it does not enhance in the arterial phase **a**. Lesion is in contact posteriorly with the right branch of the PV and anteriorly with the hepatic parenchyma of segment 4. Of note, marked dilatation of the right and left bile ducts

higher attenuation than the surrounding liver due to the abundant fibrous stroma and be better appreciated in the delayed phase (■ Fig. 5.5) [16].

Focal reduction in vessel caliber, circumferential encasement greater than 180°, and vessel occlusion are signs of vascular involvement (■ Figs. 5.6 and 5.7). The proportion of the circumferential contact between the tumor and the blood vessels or bile ducts is an important highly specificity information and should be reported among other criteria of tumor invasion (■ Table 5.4). Attenuation differences within the hepatic parenchyma surrounding the hilum are pathognomonic of parenchymal infiltration (■ Fig. 5.8).

CT reliability is limited by the presence of biliary stents, and therefore if a biliary drainage is necessary because of cholestasis, it should be placed after tumor staging has been completed. Biliary stents are radiopaque and may cause artifacts that underestimate the spread of cancer along the bile ducts. Conversely, inflammatory changes may be a consequence of drainage placement and can be misinterpreted as tumor progression along the ducts, possibly leading to overestimation.

Overall, CT is recommended as the first level test in patients with obstructive jaundice and with suspicion at ultrasound of a malignant lesion of the hepatic-pancreatic-biliary tract. However, for a more accurate assessment of horizontal spread, CT is not sufficient and needs to be integrated with *magnetic resonance cholangiopancreatography* (MRCP). MR imaging has an excellent soft

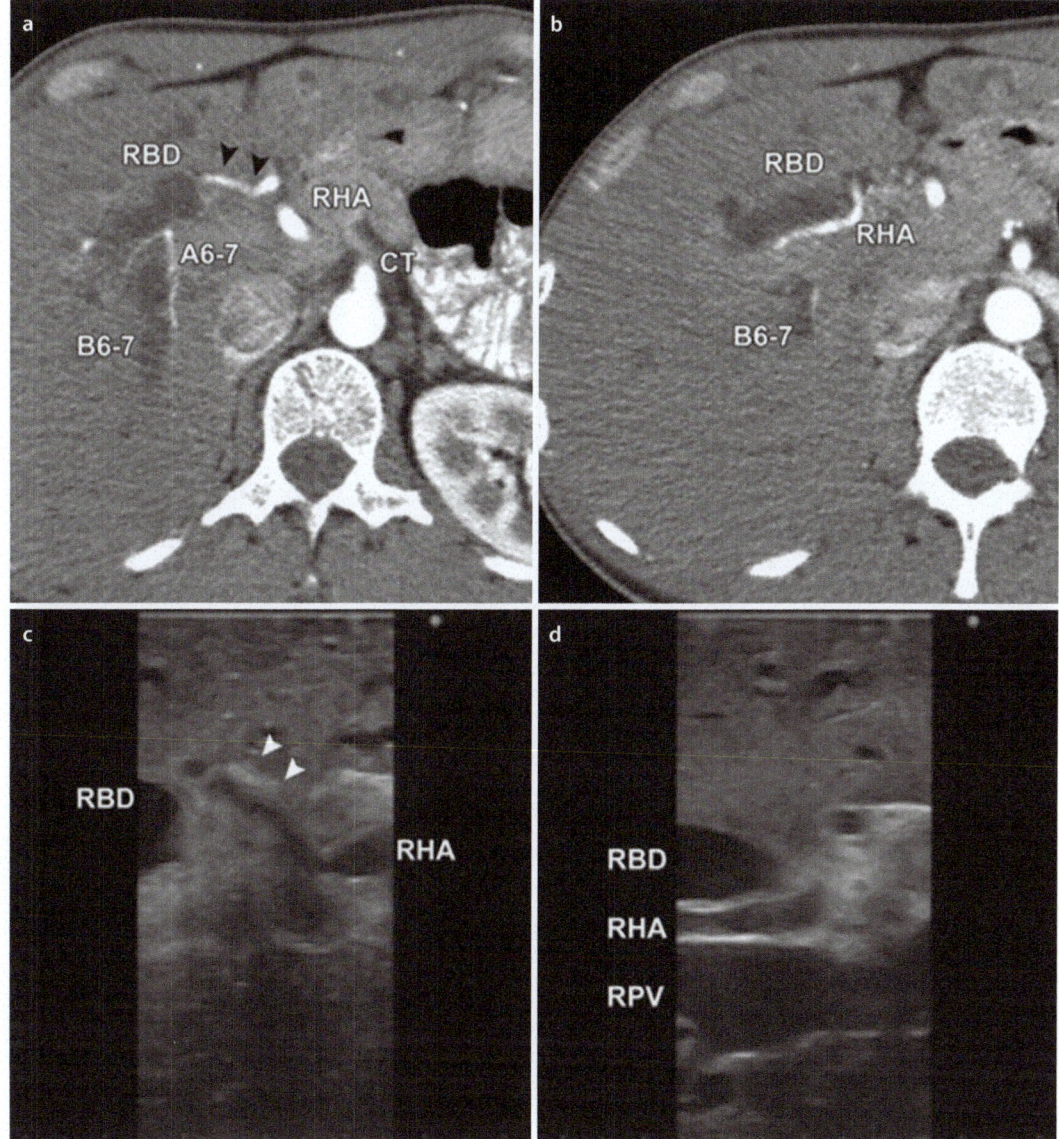

■ **Fig. 5.6** Hilar cholangiocarcinoma. **a** CT showing encasement of right hepatic artery by the tumor (*arrow points*) just before the second-order division. **b** Both the right bile duct and B6–7 are dilated. **c** Intraoperative liver ultrasound confirmed the presence and the extension of right hepatic artery infiltration (*white arrow points*) and **d** the dilatation of right bile duct. *RPV* right portal vein, *RHA* right hepatic artery, *RBD* right bile duct, *CT* celiac trunk, *B6–B7* right posterior bile duct, *A6–A7* right posterior hepatic artery

tissue contrast resolution and allows evaluation of the extent of tumor spread to the peripheral ducts, which is essential for surgical planning (■ Fig. 5.9). Compared to direct cholangiography, MRCP is noninvasive, does not require contrast medium administration, can investigate the entire biliary tree, and provides excellent quality 3D multiplanar reconstructions useful for surgical treatment planning. The use of 3D T1-weighted gradient echo sequences during intravenous administra-

tion of gadolinium chelates increases the ability to visualize vascular anatomy [18]. Combining 3D T1w dynamic sequences, performed during contrast medium administration, with MRCP, increases the diagnostic accuracy of preoperative staging with MR imaging [18–20]. Accuracy in the evaluation of bile duct involvement ranges from 81 to 96% and is more accurate for the Bismuth-Corlette type 1 and 2 hilar cholangiocarcinomas, especially when periductal or infiltrat-

5

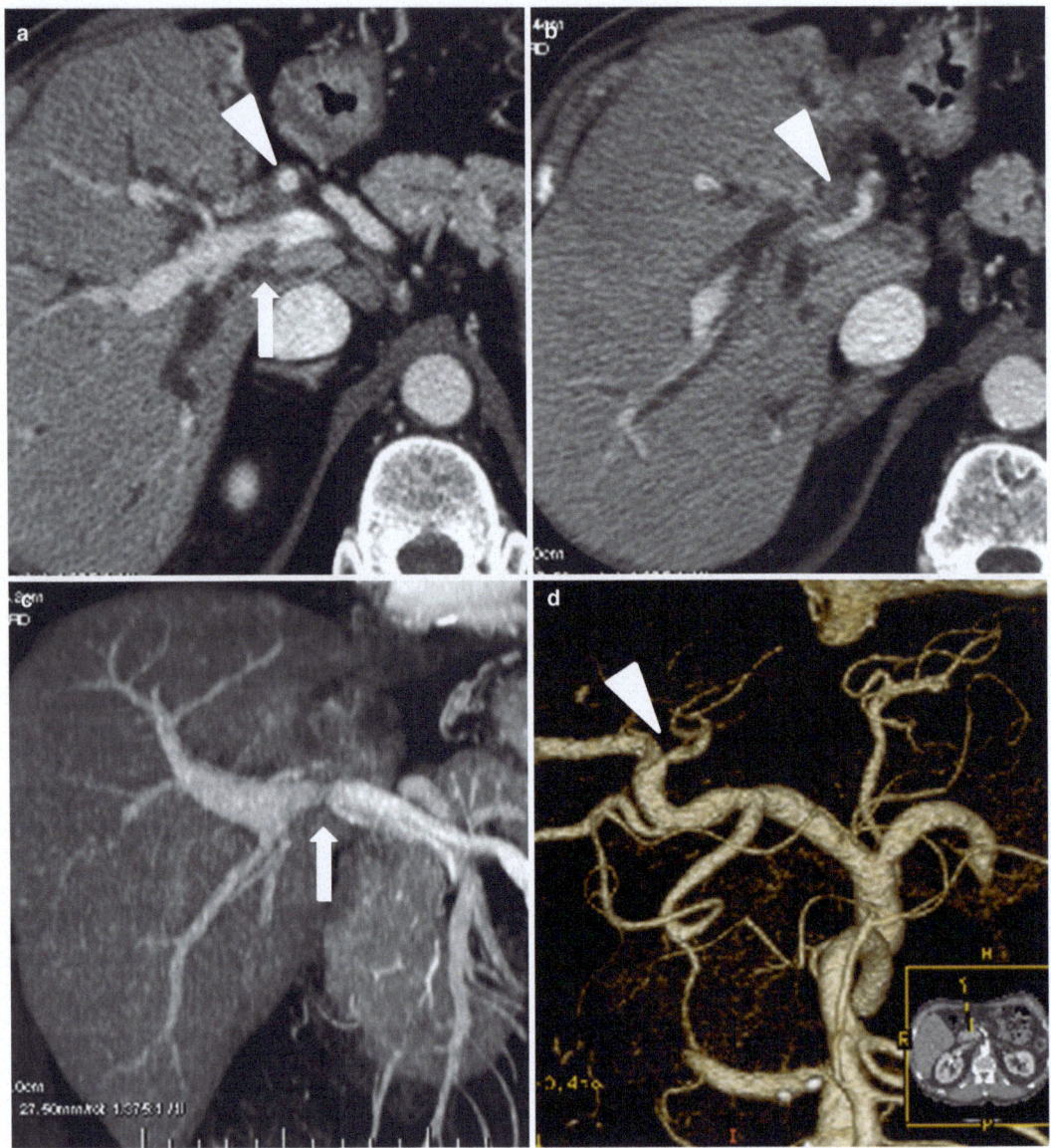

ing intraductal growth is present [16]. As for CT caution is advised if a biliary stent is present, since it can lead to an overestimation of lesion extent.

The role of FDG-PET/CT in the evaluation of hilar cholangiocarcinoma is controversial, despite most bile duct cancers being 18F-FDG avid lesions. The sensitivity of FDG-PET/CT is dependent not only on the anatomic location of the lesion but also on the growth pattern and pathologic characteristics [19]. Currently there is no clear benefit of FDG-PET/CT over CT or MRI for diagnosis or staging of the tumor, but it could be employed, in the preoperative setting, to detect metastatic spread or to differentiate between benign and malignant ambiguous lesions, while during follow up, it could allow early detection of recurrence [20].

5.1.5.2 Gallbladder Carcinoma

Gallbladder carcinoma may appear either as a mass replacing the gallbladder, as an intraluminal polyp (■ Fig. 5.10), or as a focal (■ Fig. 5.11) or

⬛ **Table 5.4** Accuracy of CT signs of vascular involvement in

Vascular infiltration parameters	Arteries		Veins	
	Sensitivity (%)	Specificity (%)	Sensitivity (%)	Specificity (%)
Incarceration or lumen obliteration	66	100	14	100
Circumferential contact > 180°	84–97	91–98	49	100
Wall irregularities	45	99	63–65	100
Stenosis	41	100	55	100

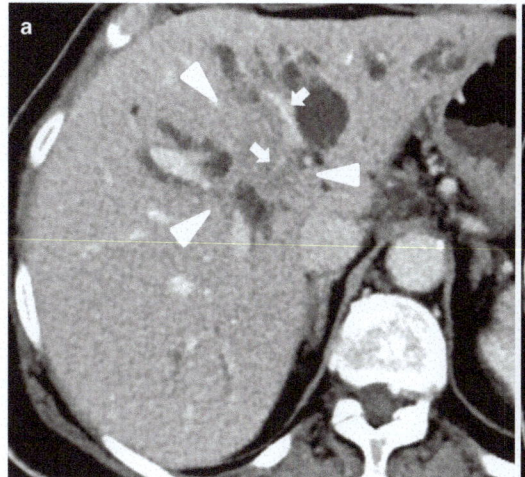

⬛ **Fig. 5.8** Extrahepatic cholangiocarcinoma. **a** Portal phase axial CT scan shows large slightly hypointense mass (*arrow points*) infiltrating the liver parenchyma in segments 1 and 4 and the right and left main portal branches (*small arrows*); **b** Delayed CT scan shows modest lesion enhancement (*arrow points*). Of note, marked dilatation of the intrahepatic bile ducts

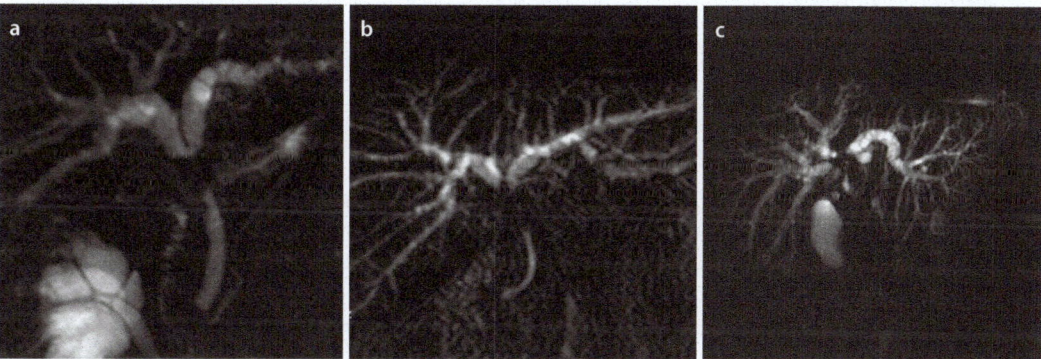

⬛ **Fig. 5.9** MRCP shows cholangiocarcinoma type I **a**, type II **b**, and type IIIa **c** according to Bismuth-Corlette classification

5

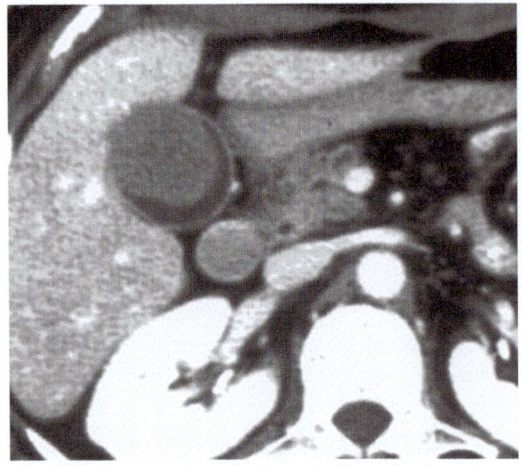

Fig. 5.10 CT scan in the venous phase shows gallbladder carcinoma with polypoid-like intraluminal growth

complete wall thickening (◘ Fig. 5.12). CT is the most used technique for the diagnosis and staging of GC [21]. The overall accuracy of CT in the identification of both the primary lesion and the local spread is reported to range between 70 and 93% [22]. CT also shows a 76% specificity and 82% sensitivity in distinguishing between malignant and benign wall thickening [23]. MR imaging shows a higher accuracy in evaluating vascular invasion (100% sensitivity, 87% specificity), bile duct involvement (68% sensitivity, 86% specificity), and hepatic invasion (90% sensitivity, 89% specificity) [23] (◘ Fig. 5.12). It also allows better differentiation between T1a and ≥T1b tumors and easier identification of gallbladder adenomyomatosis with its intramural cyst-like dilated Rokitansky-Aschoff sinuses [24]. The use of diffusion-weighted

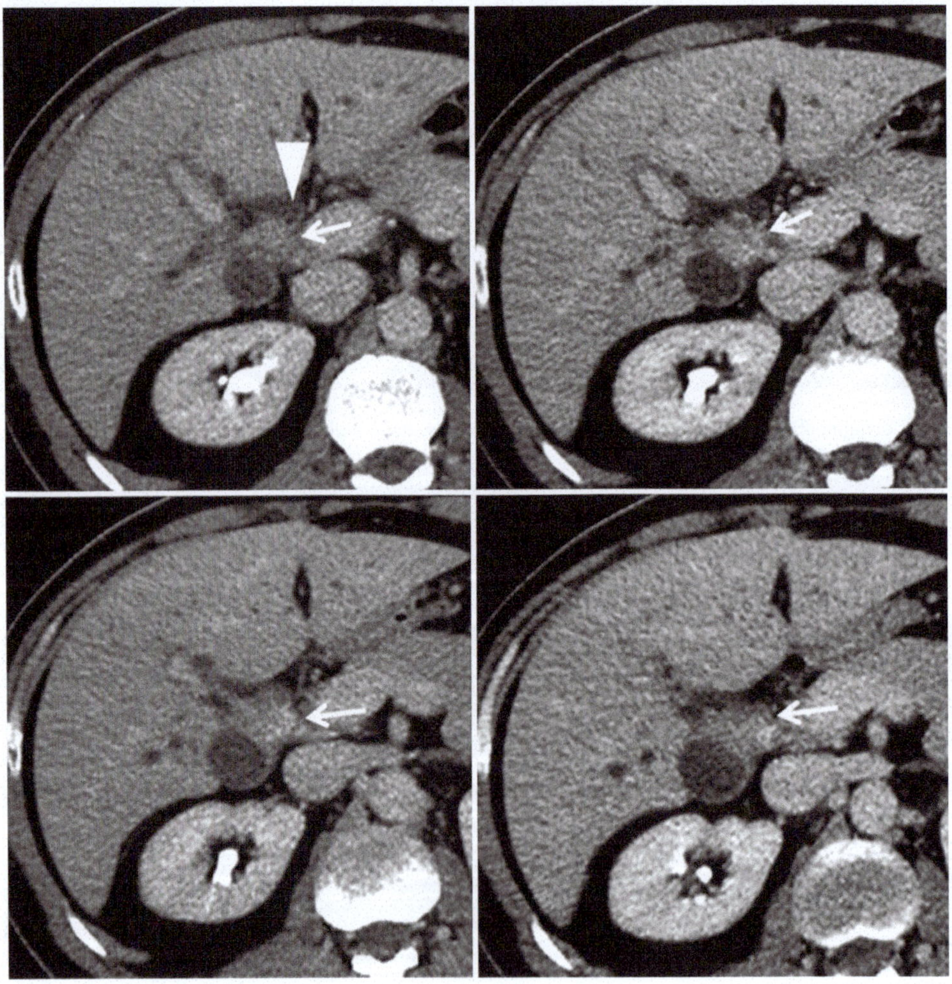

Fig. 5.11 CT scan in the delayed phase shows cholangiocarcinoma of gallbladder neck (*arrow*) infiltrating main bile duct (*arrow head*)

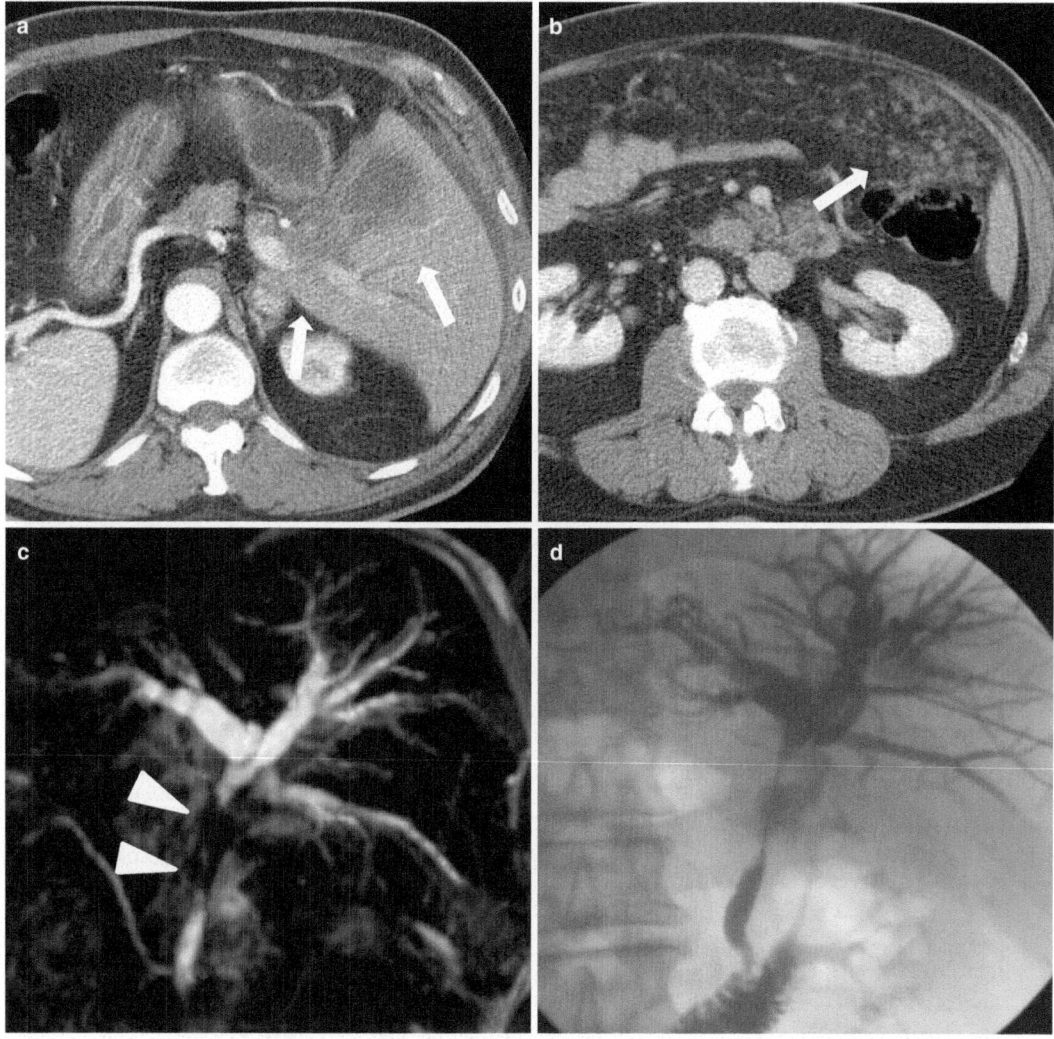

Fig. 5.12 Patient with situs inversus. **a** Axial CT scan shows a large lesion of the gallbladder infiltrating both the liver parenchyma and the hepatic pedicle (*arrows*). **b** Axial CT scan shows multiple confluent nodules of the peritoneum (*arrow*). **c** MRCP shows dilatation of intrahepatic bile ducts and stenosis of the proximal common bile duct (*arrow points*) confirmed by **d** direct cholangiography. Diagnosis of gallbladder carcinoma with peritoneal carcinomatosis

imaging (DWI) is also useful to differentiate malignant from benign lesions [22–24].

FDG-PET/CT may have a role in the preoperative assessment in the differential diagnosis of ambiguous lesions, to demonstrate distant spread and in the identification of residual disease after cholecystectomy [23].

5.1.6 Treatment

Radical resection with a microscopically negative margin (R0) is the only way to cure bile duct can-

cer and is associated with marked survival advantages. The surgical strategy is largely conditioned on the mode of tumor spread. The longitudinal spread of biliary cancers determines the type of radical operation, including extended hepatectomy and hepatopancreaticoduodenectomy. Direct invasion of major vessels, regardless of the prognosis, presents surgical challenges whose indication and operative procedures continue to be debated. When there is severe adhesion between tumor and portal vein, combined resection and reconstruction are necessary to obtain a possible negative surgical margin, yet routine

5

resection of the portal vein might not be recommended unless supported by findings from a randomized clinical trial. Distant metastasis, peritoneal carcinomatosis, and para-aortic lymph node metastasis are absolute contraindications for radical surgery in patients with biliary cancers. The criteria determining the unresectability in HC can be related to patient general status such as reduced health and cirrhosis or factors related to the extension of the disease (▶ Box 5.1) [25, 26].

> **Box 5.1   Criteria of Unresectability in Patients with Hilar Cholangiocarcinoma**
> - Bilateral extension to the second biliary confluence with bilateral hepatic artery or portal vein invasion
> - Invasion of the main trunk of the portal vein (before its bifurcation) or hepatic artery
> - Atrophy of a liver lobe with contralateral vascular invasion or extension to the contralateral second biliary branch
> - Unilateral extension of the tumor to the sectional bile ducts with involvement of the contralateral portal vein
> - Metastasis to the para-aortic lymph nodes
> - Distant metastases

The role of cytotoxic therapy for advanced biliary cancer remains controversial because of the minimal impact on the disease. Gemcitabine alone or in combination with cisplatin or oxaliplatin is the most commonly used agents for advanced-stage biliary cancer. Combination chemotherapy might improve response rates but is indicated only for patients with a good performance status due to the higher toxicity [27]. The association of chemotherapeutic agents and precision radiation techniques may improve local control and survival in patients with advanced biliary cancer [28].

5.1.7   Prognosis

Median overall survival rate is low, since most patients are not eligible for curative resection. Extrahepatic bile duct cancer shows a 5-year survival rate of 30% in patients with localized disease, 24% if regional spread is present, and 2% for those with distant localizations [15–17].

5.2   Patterns of Local Spread and Implications to Treatment

5.2.1   Local Spread of Gallbladder Carcinoma

Gallbladder carcinoma spreads early on in its course usually by direct liver extension. Anatomy facilitates spread to the liver. Indeed, the gallbladder wall lacks a submucosal layer, and no serosa is present where the viscera are attached to the liver. Consequently, the tumor invades through the thin gallbladder wall early and then extends directly to the liver (around the gallbladder fossa) and adjacent structures, mainly the bile duct (◘ Fig. 5.12).

Surgical approach is strictly dependent on T stage. Tis/T1a gallbladder cancer is typically diagnosed after cholecystectomy for lithiasis and requires no further treatment [29]. Wedge resection of the gallbladder bed or bisegmentectomy S4b-5 and N1 lymph node dissection are recommended in the treatment of T1b and T2 disease [30]. Conversely, the treatment of a locally advanced carcinoma of the gallbladder T3/T4 remains a challenge [31]. Overall, patient survival is higher when only major hepatectomy is performed than when pancreatoduodenectomy or resection of other organs is needed [32].

5.2.2   Local Spread of Hilar Cholangiocarcinoma

Hilar cholangiocarcinoma spreads locally by transmural invasion of the bile duct wall. Cancer may spread longitudinally along the right and left hepatic ducts but also disseminate in the cranial and dorsal directions along the thin lateral bile ducts. It is common for HC to infiltrate the hepatic parenchyma and the hepatoduodenal ligament. In particular, HC may extend anteriorly to involve the base of segment 4 or extend in posteriorly to the short bile ducts of the caudate lobe. The main goal of surgical resection in patients with HC is to remove the liver parenchyma adjacent to the hepatic hilum together with the hilar plate to achieve a complete curative resection. In this sense, complete caudate lobectomy and resection of the inferior part of Couinaud's segment 4 coupled with right or left hemihepatectomy (according to the

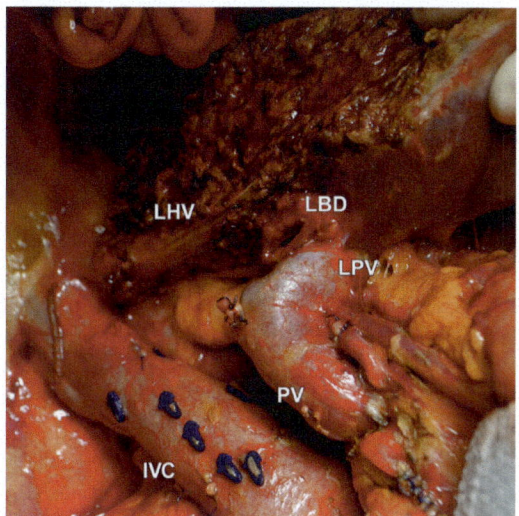

Right trisectionectomy extended to segment 1, bile duct resection, and lymphadenectomy for right-side hilar cholangiocarcinoma. *IVC* inferior vena cava, *LHV* left hepatic vein, *LBD* left bile duct, *LPV* left portal vein, *PV* portal vein

predominant tumor location) are the gold standard treatments of HC. Generally an extended right hemihepatectomy is preferentially indicated for even centrally located tumors, because of the greater length of left hepatic duct that facilitates the goal of the negative margin [33] (■ Fig. 5.13). The pattern of infiltration at the proximal border of HC closely relates to the gross tumor type [34]. The papillary type has a predominantly intraluminal growth pattern. By contrast, the nodular infiltrative or sclerosing gross types spread longitudinally along the duct wall but also present with microscopic intramural extension. Superficial spread, defined as a mucosal extension of more than 20 mm, is observed in more than 10% of hilar cholangiocarcinomas, more frequently in the papillary and well-differentiated types [35–37]. A gross surgical margin of more than 1 cm in the infiltrating type, and of more than 2 cm in the papillary and nodular types, is recommended to obtain microscopically negative margins.

5.3 Vessel Infiltration and Resectability

The right hepatic artery runs just behind the common hepatic duct, and the portal bifurcation is located very close to the confluence of the hepatic ducts. These anatomical considerations justify the high rate of vascular infiltration in patients with biliary cancer. Commonly, invasion of the portal vein walls proceeds from the adventitia to the intima. In other cases, following endothelial destruction, a thrombus may form and progress until the lumen of the vein is totally obliterated. When there is severe adhesion between the tumor and portal vein, combined resection and reconstruction are necessary to obtain negative surgical margins [38, 39].

Invasion of the right hepatic artery may be the consequence of direct extension of the tumor to the hepatoduodenal ligament or may be secondary to the infiltration of the hepatic pedicle by a lymph node metastasis. With the advances in surgical technique, it is now possible to perform hepatic artery resection and reconstruction; however, the true benefit in terms of survival for this aggressive approach is yet to be established [40].

5.4 Involvement of Adjacent Organs

Duodenum, colon, and other abdominal viscera may be directly invaded by biliary cancer. In the absence of distant metastases, the involvement of adjacent organs does not constitute per se a criterion for non-resectability. Combination of hepatectomy and pancreaticoduodenectomy is commonly indicated when there is direct duodenal or pancreatic invasion and peripancreatic lymph node involvement [41]. The survival benefits of these procedures remain unclear; consequently this aggressive surgery is not routinely recommended.

5.5 Lymph Node Involvement

5.5.1 Gallbladder Carcinoma

Ito and Mishima divided the lymphatic drainage of the gallbladder into the following three pathways based on detailed dissections of the lymphatic system of adult cadavers: the cholecysto-retropancreatic, the cholecystocoeliac, and the cholecysto-mesenteric pathway. These three pathways converge with the abdominal aortic lymph nodes near the left renal vein. Recently, Wakay et al.

5

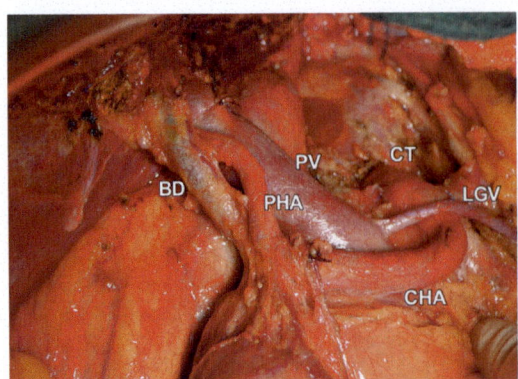

☐ **Fig. 5.14** Operative field after N2-lymphadenectomy in the treatment of gallbladder carcinoma. *PV* portal vein, *LGV* left gastric vein, *CT* celiac trunk, *CHA* common hepatic artery, *PHA* proper hepatic artery, *BD* bile duct

[15] have shown, thanks to immunohistochemical analysis, that portal tract invasion mainly results from lymphatic spread within the portal tracts. The frequency of lymph node involvement is strongly influenced by the depth of invasion of the GC. Regional lymph node metastases occur in 19–62% and 75–85% of patients with T2 and T3/T4 GC, respectively [42]. Based on the lymphatic spread pathways and the frequency of regional N1 and N2 lymph node involvement, regional lymph node dissection is indicated in T2 and T3/T4 stage GC (☐ Fig. 5.14). The role of para-aortic lymph node dissection in advanced GC is not known. Kondo et al. showed that postoperative survival for patients with positive para-aortic lymph nodes without distant metastases was as poor as those patients with distant metastases [43].

5.5.2 Hilar Cholangiocarcinoma

Lymphatic metastases from HC appear to spread first to the pericholedochal nodes in the hepatoduodenal ligament and then to spread widely toward the posterosuperior area around the pancreatic head, portal vein, and common hepatic artery [41, 42]. The para-aortic nodes are regarded as the final nodes in the abdominal lymphatic system from the bile duct. In patients with hilar cholangiocarcinoma, N1 and N2 regional lymph node dissection is indicated. Patients with nodal involvement beyond the hepatoduodenal ligament, including para-aortic nodal metastases, were shown to have dismal prognosis with a 5-year survival of 0–12%. Therefore, routine

lymph node dissection beyond the hepatoduodenal ligament is not recommended.

5.6 Perineural Invasion

Perineural invasion can occur by direct invasion of peribiliary nerve plexus and/or via perineural lymphatic vessels. This phenomenon seems to be highly correlated with tumor volume, location, depth of invasiveness, angiogenesis, and lymph node involvement. It has been shown that perineural invasion is correlated with neural cell adhesion molecules (NCAM) expression, indicating that NCAM molecules on the surface of tumor cells might induce them to migrate and adhere to nerve cells when the tumor breaches their capsule. Perineural invasion in advanced GC is strictly associated to extrahepatic biliary infiltration [44, 45], and it represents an independent pathway of spread into the liver.

5.7 Metastatic Spread

Hematogenous spread of biliary cancer occurs most commonly to the liver and the peritoneum (☐ Fig. 5.12). Metastases to other organs, such as the lungs, osseous structures, kidneys, adrenals, and brain, occur less frequently. Diagnostic laparoscopy at the time of operation identifies unresectable or metastatic disease in ~50% of patients with gallbladder cancer [46]. There are a number of factors that may contribute to gallbladder cancer spread into the peritoneum such as the anatomical location of the gallbladder that has relations inferiorly with the peritoneal surfaces and the immobility of the omental bursa, which promotes a gravitational distribution of tumor cells and the intrinsic characteristics of the peritoneum. Indeed, the microenvironment of peritoneum is hypoxic, well vascularized, and lined with mesothelium overlaying immune aggregates, which express pro-angiogenic and adhesion molecules that are highly selective for tumor growth and evolution [44].

References

1. Blechacz BR, Gores GJ (2008) Cholangiocarcinoma. Clin Liver Dis 12(1):131–150. ix
2. Chung YE et al (2009) Varying appearances of cholangiocarcinoma: radiologic-pathologic correlation. Radiographics 29(3):683–700

3. Bile Duct Cancer (Cholangiocarcinoma), American Cancer Society (2016) http://www.cancer.org/cancer/bileductcancer/

4. Hsing AW, Rashid A, Devesa SS et al (2006) Biliary tract cancer. In: Cancer epidemiology and prevention, 3rd edn. Oxford University Press, New York, pp 878–900

5. Khan SA et al (2008) Epidemiology, risk factors, and pathogenesis of cholangiocarcinoma. HPB 10:77–82

6. Abou-Alfa GK, Jarnagin W, Lowery M et al (2014) Chapter 80: liver and bile duct cancer. In: Abeloff's clinical oncology, 5th edn. Elsevier, Philadelphia

7. Thomas CR, Fuller CD (2008) Biliary tract and gallbladder cancer: diagnosis & therapy. Demosmedical, New York

8. Herma JM et al (2008) Biliary tract and gallbladder cancer: a multidisciplinary approach, 2nd edn. Demosmedical, New York

9. Nakanuma Y, Kakuda Y (2015) Pathologic classification of cholangiocarcinoma: new concepts. Best Pract Res Clin Gastroenterol 29:277–293

10. Wan X-S, Xu Y-Y, Qian J-Y et al (2013) Intraductal papillary neoplasm of the bile duct. World J Gastroenterol 19(46):8595–8604

11. American Joint Committee on Cancer (2010) AJCC cancer staging manual, 7th edn. Springer, New York, pp 201–205. 219–230

12. Ruys AT et al (2013) Prognostic impact of preoperative imaging parameters on resectability of hilar cholangiocarcinoma. HPB Surg 2013:657309

13. Suarez-Munoz MA et al (2013) Risk factors and classifications of hilar cholangiocarcinoma. World J Gastrointest Oncol 5(7):132–138

14. Blechacz BR et al (2011) Clinical diagnosis and staging of cholangiocarcinoma. Nat Rev Gastroenterol Hepatol 8(9):512–522

15. Wakai T, Shirai Y, Moroda T, Yokoyama N, Hatakeyama K (2005) Impact of ductal resection margin status on long-term survival in patients undergoing resection for extrahepatic cholangiocarcinoma. Cancer 103(6):1210–1216

16. Vogel A et al (2014) The diagnosis and treatment of cholangiocarcinoma. Dtsch Arztebl Int 111(44): 748–754

17. Mansour JC et al (2015) Hilar cholangiocarcinoma: expert consensus statement. HPB (Oxford) 17(8): 691–699

18. Vilgrain V (2008) Staging cholangiocarcinoma by imaging studies. HPB 10:106–109

19. Choi JI et al (2008) Hilar cholangiocarcinoma: role of preoperative imaging with sonography, MDCT, MRI, and direct cholangiography. AJR Am J Roentgenol 191(5):1448–1457

20. Cui XY et al (2012) Diffusion-weighted MR imaging for detection of extrahepatic cholangiocarcinoma. Eur J Radiol 81(11):2961–2965

21. Ringe KI, Wacker F (2015) Radiological diagnosis in cholangiocarcinoma: application of computed tomography, magnetic resonance imaging, and positron emission tomography. Best Pract Res Clin Gastroenterol 29(2):253–265. https://doi.org/10.1016/j.bpg.2015.02.004. Epub 2015 Feb 17

22. Chung YE et al (2008) Staging of extrahepatic cholangiocarcinoma. Eur Radiol 18:2182–2195. https://doi.org/10.1007/s00330-008-1006-x

23. Kanthan R et al (2015) Gallbladder cancer in the 21st century. J Oncol 2015:967472

24. Lai CH, Lau WY (2008) Gallbladder cancer-a comprehensive review. Surgeon 6(2):101–110

25. Russolillo N, D'Eletto M, Langella S, Perotti S, Lo Tesoriere R, Forchino F, Ferrero A (2016) Role of laparoscopic ultrasound during diagnostic laparoscopy for proximal biliary cancers: a single series of 100 patients. Surg Endosc 30(3):1212–1218

26. Jarnagin WR, Bowne W, Klimstra DS, Ben-Porat L, Roggin K, Cymes K, Fong Y, DeMatteo RP, D'Angelica M, Koea J, Blumgart LH (2005) Papillary phenotype confers improved survival after resection of hilar cholangiocarcinoma. Ann Surg 241(5):703–712. discussion 712–4

27. Valle JW, Wasan HS, Palmer DD et al (2009) Gemcitabine with or without cisplatin in patients (PTS) with advanced or metastatic biliary tract cancer (ABC): results of a multicenter, randomized phase III trial (the UK ABC-02 trial). Proc Am Soc Clin Oncol 27:4503–4503

28. Wang SJ, Lemieux A, Kalpathy-Cramer J et al (2011) Nomogram for predicting the benefit of adjuvant chemoradiotherapy for resected gallbladder cancer. J Clin Oncol 29(35):4627–4632

29. Sakamoto E, Nimura Y, Hayakawa N, Kamiya J, Kondo S, Nagino M, Kanai M, Miyachi M, Uesaka K (1998) The pattern of infiltration at the proximal border of hilar bile duct carcinoma: a histologic analysis of 62 resected cases. Ann Surg 227(3):405–411

30. Kitagawa Y, Nagino M, Kamiya J, Uesaka K, Sano T, Yamamoto H, Hayakawa N, Nimura Y (2001) Lymph node metastasis from hilar cholangiocarcinoma: audit of 110 patients who underwent regional and paraaortic node dissection. Ann Surg 233(3):385–392

31. Endo I et al (2007) Role of three-dimensional imaging in operative planning for hilar cholangiocarcinoma. Surgery 142(5):666–675

32. Nimura Y, Kamiya J, Kondo S, Nagino M, Uesaka K, Oda K, Sano T, Yamamoto H, Hayakawa N (2000) Aggressive preoperative management and extended surgery for hilar cholangiocarcinoma: nagoya experience. J Hepato-Biliary-Pancreat Surg 7(2):155–162

33. Goetze TO, Paolucci V (2008) Benefits of reoperation of T2 and more advanced incidental gallbladder carcinoma: analysis of the German registry. Ann Surg 247(1):104–108

34. Muratore A, Bouzari H, Polastri R, Vergara V, Capussotti L (2000) Radical surgery for gallbladder cancer: a worthwhile operation? Eur J Surg Oncol 26(2):160–163

35. Birnbaum DJ, Viganò L, Ferrero A, Langella S, Russolillo N, Capussotti L (2014) Locally advanced gallbladder cancer: which patients benefit from resection? Eur J Surg Oncol 40(8):1008–1015

36. Sasaki R, Takahashi M, Funato O et al (2002) Hepatopancreatoduodenectomy with wide lymph node dissection for locally advanced carcinoma of the gallbladder e long-term results. Hepato-Gastroenterology 49:912–915

5

37. Birnbaum DJ, Viganò L, Russolillo N, Langella S, Ferrero A, Capussotti L (2015) Lymph node metastases in patients undergoing surgery for a gallbladder cancer. Extension of the lymph node dissection and prognostic value of the lymph node ratio. Ann Surg Oncol 22(3):811–818

38. Kondo S, Katoh H, Hirano S, Ambo Y, Tanaka E, Okushiba S (2003) Portal vein resection and reconstruction prior to hepatic dissection during right hepatectomy and caudate lobectomy for hepatobiliary cancer. Br J Surg 90(6):694–697

39. Nimura Y, Hayakawa N, Kamiya J, Maeda S, Kondo S, Yasui A, Shionoya S, Goetze TO, Paolucci V (2008) Immediate re-resection of T1 incidental gallbladder carcinomas: a survival analysis of the German Registry. Surg Endosc 22(11):2462–2465

40. Ebata T, Nagino M, Kamiya J, Uesaka K, Nagasaka T, Nimura Y (2003) Hepatectomy with portal vein resection for hilar cholangiocarcinoma: audit of 52 consecutive cases. Ann Surg 238(5):720–727

41. Hirano S, Kondo S, Tanaka E, Shichinohe T, Tsuchikawa T, Kato K (2009) No-touch resection of hilar malignancies with right hepatectomy and routine portal reconstruction. J Hepato-Biliary-Pancreat Surg 16(4):502–507. Epub 2009 Apr 10

42. Nagino M, Nimura Y, Nishio H, Ebata T, Igami T, Matsushita M, Nishikimi N, Kamei Y (2010) Hepatectomy with simultaneous resection of the portal vein and hepatic artery for advanced perihilar cholangiocarcinoma: an audit of 50 consecutive cases. Ann Surg 252(1): 115–123

43. Duraker N, Sisman S, Can G (2003) The significance of perineural invasion as a prognostic factor in patients with gastric carcinoma. Surg Today 33:95–100

44. Murakawa K, Tada M, Takada M, Tamoto E, Shindoh G, Teramoto K et al (2004) Prediction of lymph node metastasis and perineural invasion of biliary tract cancer by selected features from cDNA array data. J Surg Res 122:184–194

45. Shen F-Z, Zhang B-Y, Feng Y-J, Jia Z-X, An B, Liu C-C, Deng X-Y, Kulkarni AD, Lu Y (2010) Current research in perineural invasion of cholangiocarcinoma. J Exp Clin Cancer Res 29(1):24

46. Maplanka C (2014) Gallbladder cancer, treatment failure and relapses: the peritoneum in gallbladder cancer. J Gastrointest Cancer 45(3):2

Pancreatic Adenocarcinoma

Giulia Zamboni, Maria Chiara Ambrosetti, Laura Maggino, and Giuseppe Malleo

© Springer International Publishing AG 2018
D. Regge, G. Zamboni (eds.), *Hepatobiliary and Pancreatic Cancer,*
Cancer Dissemination Pathways, https://doi.org/10.1007/978-3-319-50296-0_6

6.1 Overview

6.1.1 Epidemiology

The American Cancer Society estimates that about 48,960 new cases of pancreatic cancer (24,840 in men and 24,120 in women) will be diagnosed in the USA in 2015 [1]. The overall incidence of pancreatic cancer has been relatively stable for decades.

Although pancreatic cancer constitutes only about 3% of all cancers in the USA, it accounts for about 7% of all cancer-related deaths, being the fourth leading cause of cancer deaths in both men and women [2].

6.1.2 Risk Factors

Estimates indicate that 40% of pancreatic cancer cases are sporadic in nature, up to 30% are related to smoking, and 20% may be associated with dietary factors. Only 5–10% are hereditary in nature [3].

Diabetes mellitus increases the risk for pancreatic adenocarcinoma. The National Comprehensive Cancer Network (NCCN) guideline for pancreatic adenocarcinoma (2.2011 version) acknowledges long-standing diabetes mellitus as a risk factor for pancreatic cancer.

Another important risk factor is chronic pancreatitis: the risk increases linearly with time, with 4% of patients who had chronic pancreatitis for 20 years duration developing pancreatic cancer.

The risk is even higher in patients with hereditary pancreatitis (increased more than 50-fold).

6.1.3 Pathology

Ductal adenocarcinoma arises from, and is phenotypically similar to, pancreatic duct epithelium, with mucin production and expression of a characteristic cytokeratin pattern.

Most ductal adenocarcinomas are well to moderately differentiated. They usually consist of well-developed glandular structures, which more or less imitate normal pancreatic ducts, embedded in a fibrous desmoplastic stroma.

It is the most common tumor in the pancreas, accounting for 85–90% of all pancreatic neoplasms. The majority (approximately 75%) arise in the head of the pancreas, mainly in the upper half, less commonly in the uncinate process, 15–20% in the body, and 5–10% in the pancreatic tail.

Ductal adenocarcinomas are firm and poorly defined masses. Hemorrhage and necrosis are uncommon, while microcystic areas may be present.

The pancreas is anatomically divided into three main parts: head, body, and tail. The head of the pancreas includes the neck (anterior to the superior mesenteric vein and the portal vein) and the uncinate process. The boundary between the head and body of the pancreas is the left margin of the superior mesenteric and portal vein. Body and tail of the pancreas are collectively referred to as distal pancreas; the boundary between body and tail is the line dividing the distal pancreas into two equal halves.

Given the different characteristics of lymphvascular and neural stream and the distinctive relationship with the contiguous organs, tumors originating from each portion of the pancreas display a peculiar behavior in terms of local invasion.

The identification of such specific patterns of tumor spread in relation to the site of origin within the gland is of paramount importance in guiding surgical decision-making as regards both the assessment of resectability and the definition of the optimal extension of the resection.

6.1.4 Staging

The evaluation of the extent of local invasion is fundamental for tumor staging, in order to identify patients who are eligible for resection with curative intent. The preferred staging system for pancreatic cancers is the tumor-node-metastasis (TNM) system of the combined American Joint Committee on Cancer (AJCC)/International Union Against Cancer (UICC). In this classification, the characteristics of local aggressiveness are taken into account both in the evaluation of the T and N parameters (◻ Tables 6.1 and 6.2).

6.1.5 Treatment

Treatment of pancreatic cancer depends on the stage of the disease, dividing patients with resectable, locally advanced (unresectable) or metastatic disease.

▣ Table 6.1 TNM staging for pancreatic carcinoma

Primary tumor (T)	
TX	Primary tumor cannot be assessed
T0	No evidence of primary tumor
Tis	Carcinoma in situ
T1	Tumor limited to the pancreas, ≤2 cm in greatest dimension
T2	Tumor limited to the pancreas, >2 cm in greatest dimension
T3	Tumor extends beyond the pancreas but without involvement of the celiac axis or the superior mesenteric artery
T4	Tumor involves the celiac axis or the superior mesenteric artery (unresectable primary tumor)
Regional lymph nodes (N)	
NX	Regional lymph nodes cannot be assessed
N0	No regional lymph node metastasis
N1	Regional lymph node metastasis
Distant metastasis (M)	
M0	No distant metastasis
M1	Distant metastasis

▣ Table 6.2 Stage grouping for pancreatic cancer

Stage	
0	Tis, N0, M0
IA	T1, N0, M0
IB	T2, N0, M0
IIA	T3, N0, M0
IIB	T1-3, N1, M0
III	T4, Any N, M0
IV	Any T, Any N, M1

Patients with resectable cancer should undergo upfront surgery; depending on tumor location, this can be pancreaticoduodenectomy, distal pancreatectomy, or total pancreatectomy.

Chemotherapy may be used in neoadjuvant regimens, for adjuvant postoperative therapy, or as a single treatment in metastatic patients.

Medical treatment of metastatic pancreatic cancer is based on both FOLFIRINOX [4] and administration of gemcitabine and nabpaclitaxel [5].

Performance status, assessment of comorbidities, and presence of biliary stents are the main criteria for the choice of treatment.

6.1.6 Prognosis

Overall 5-year survival rate is 7.2%, ranging from 27.1% for localized disease to 2.4% for metastatic disease (▣ Tables 6.3 and 6.4).

▣ Table 6.3 5-Year observed survival rate (%)

Stage	5-Year observed survival rate (%)
IA	14
IB	12
IIA	7
IIB	5
III	3
IV	1

▣ Table 6.4 5-Year relative survival (%) for 2005–2011 (SEER Cancer Statistic Review)

Stage at diagnosis	Both sexes	Males	Females
All stages	7.2	7.0	7.3
Localized	27.1	27.0	27.0
Regional	10.7	11.1	10.3
Distant	2.4	2.4	2.5
Unstaged	4.4	5.0	4.0

6.2 Patterns of Local Spread

6.2.1 Introduction

Besides its well-known metastatic aptitude, pancreatic ductal adenocarcinoma (PDAC) is characterized by a striking tendency for loco-regional dissemination. Local extension of the tumor is determined by multiple factors, reflecting both the peculiar biology of the cancer cells and the complexity of the anatomical location of the pancreas. The dense network of nerves, blood vessels, and lymphatic vessels surrounding the gland constitutes the optimal basis for tumor's local infiltration and involvement of adjacent organs that often occurs.

When the tumor is located mainly in the head of the pancreas, vascular invasion often occurs in the portal/superior mesenteric axis (◘ Fig. 6.1a). Conversely, when the tumor is located in the body and tail of the pancreas, it generally infiltrates the celiac trunk and/or the splenic vessels [6] (◘ Fig. 6.1b).

Occasionally, local invasion may also involve the inferior vena cava (especially for tumors arising in the pancreatic head) or, rarely, the aorta (tumors of the pancreatic head or body). The degree of vascular involvement is a fundamental parameter in cancer staging, and vascular invasion is the main determinant of local resectability [7].

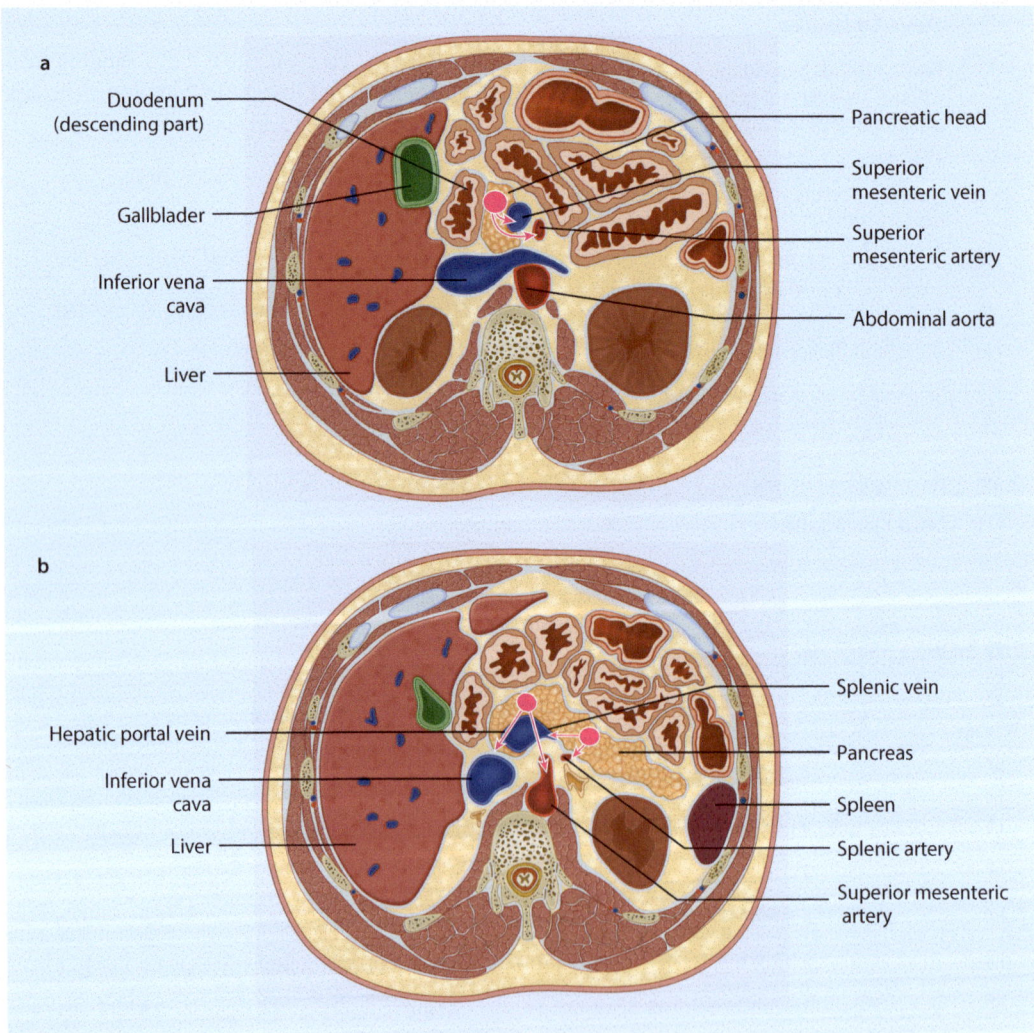

◘ **Fig. 6.1**   Anatomy and spread patterns to the vessels for tumors in the pancreatic head **a** and body/tail **b**

6.3 Vessel Infiltration and Resectability

Given the absence of distant metastases, a tumor is considered resectable when clear fat planes can be identified around the celiac axis, hepatic artery, and superior mesenteric artery, and there is no radiologic evidence of superior mesenteric vein or portal vein distortion (◘ Fig. 6.2).

The term "borderline resectable pancreatic cancer" (BRPC) is commonly used to describe tumors involving the porto-mesenteric or arterial axis, that is, an intermediate stage between straightforwardly resectable and technically unresectable disease.

The concept of borderline resectable itself is continuously evolving, in relation with the improvement of operative techniques and the deepening of the knowledge on the impact of vascular resections in terms of morbidity, mortality, and long-term survival.

As such, in the latest version of the NCCN guidelines (2015.2) the definition of BRPC has been reformulated (◘ Table 6.5) and slight differences from the ISGPS consensus statement [8] have been introduced.

The definition of unresectability is related to the location of the primary tumor (◘ Table 6.6).

For all tumor sites, tumors are considered unresectable if there are distant metastases, or LN metastases beyond the field of resection.

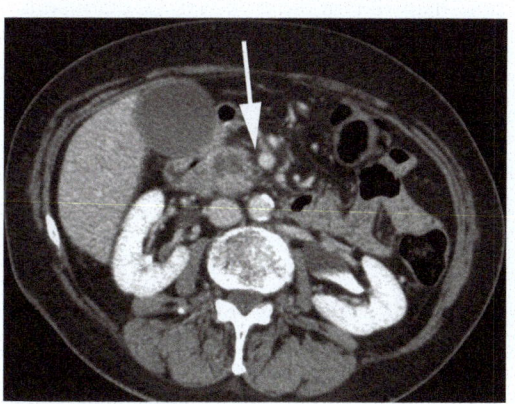

◘ **Fig. 6.2** Resectable tumor, a fat plane is seen between the tumor and the mesenteric vessels (*arrow*)

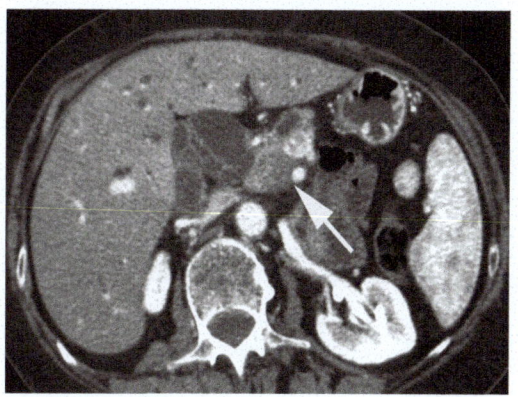

◘ **Fig. 6.3** 180° encasement of the SMA (*arrow*)—borderline resectable pancreatic cancer (BRPC)

◘ Table 6.5 2015 NCCN guidelines, definition of BRPC tumors	
Tumors in the head/ uncinate process	Contact with the common hepatic artery without extension to celiac axis or hepatic artery bifurcation, allowing for safe and complete resection/reconstruction
	Tumor contact with the SMA ≤180° (◘ Fig. 6.3)
	Presence of variant anatomy, and the presence/degree of tumor contact should be noted because it may affect surgical planning
Distal tumors	Contact with celiac axis of ≤180°
	Contact with celiac axis of >180° without involvement of the aorta and with intact and uninvolved gastroduodenal artery
All locations	Contact with SMV or PV of >180°, contact of ≤180° with contour irregularity or thrombosis of the vein but with suitable vessel proximal and distal to the site of involvement, allowing for safe and complete resection/reconstruction (◘ Fig. 6.4)
	Contact with the inferior vena cava

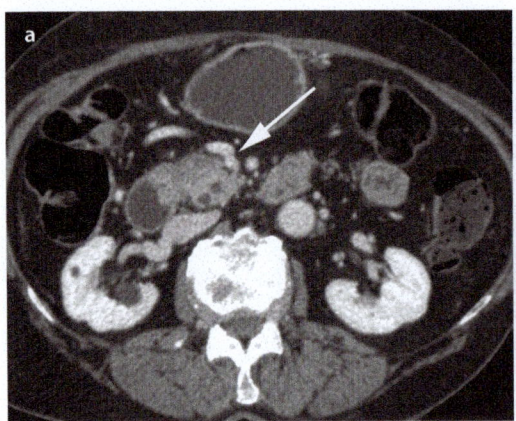 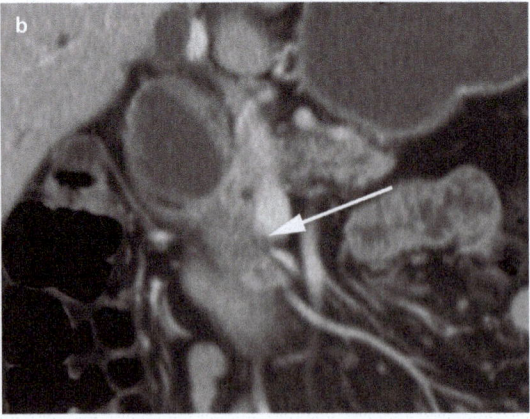

☐ **Fig. 6.4** Axial **a** and coronal **b** CT images show a short contact between tumor and SMV (*arrow* in **a** and **b**), therefore defining a BRPC

6

☐ **Table 6.6**	Definition of unresectability
Tumor site	**Criteria for unresectability**
Head of pancreas	>180° superior mesenteric artery encasement, any celiac abutment (☐ Fig. 6.5)
	Non-reconstructable superior mesenteric/portal vein occlusion (☐ Figs. 6.6, 6.7, and 6.8)
	Aortic or inferior vena cava invasion or encasement
Body of pancreas	Superior mesenteric artery or celiac encasement >180° (☐ Fig. 6.9)
	Non-reconstructable superior mesenteric/portal vein occlusion
	Aortic invasion or encasement
Tail of pancreas	Superior mesenteric artery or celiac encasement >180°
For all sites	Distant metastases (☐ Figs. 6.10 and 6.11)
	Metastases to lymph nodes beyond the field of resection

Tumors in the head of the pancreas are considered straightforwardly unresectable if the superior mesenteric artery is encased for more than 180°, if there is any abutment of the celiac axis, if there is invasion of the aorta or the inferior vena cava, or if there is a non-reconstructable occlusion of the superior mesenteric vein or the portal vein.

Tumors in the body of the pancreas are considered unresectable if there is encasement for more than 180° of the celiac axis or the superior mesenteric vein, invasion or encasement of the aorta, or a non-reconstructable occlusion of the superior mesenteric vein or the portal vein.

Tumors in the tail of the pancreas are unresectable when they encase for >180° the celiac axis or the superior mesenteric artery.

6.3.1 Splenic Vessels Infiltration

Splenic vessels constitute a relatively frequent site of local invasion by tumors arising in the distal pancreas: the rate of splenic artery and vein invasion in resected PDAC is reported around 20–30% and 50%, respectively [6, 9].

Surgical resection is commonly performed if infiltration of both the splenic vein and artery (T3 category) is present.

Retrospective studies on patients undergoing distal pancreatectomy [6, 9] have demonstrated that splenic artery infiltration is an independent predictor of survival, while splenic vein invasion is not. This might be explained based on anatomic considerations: the splenic artery courses a few millimeters outside the pancreas, whereas the splenic vein runs within the gland (☐ Fig. 6.12). Arterial invasion could therefore represent an indicator of extrapancreatic tumor spread. In addition, given that pancreatic cancer is known to metastasize via the axonal flow, the dense network of nerves that surrounds the splenic artery could facilitate tumor progression upstream to the celiac plexus, leading to adverse prognosis.

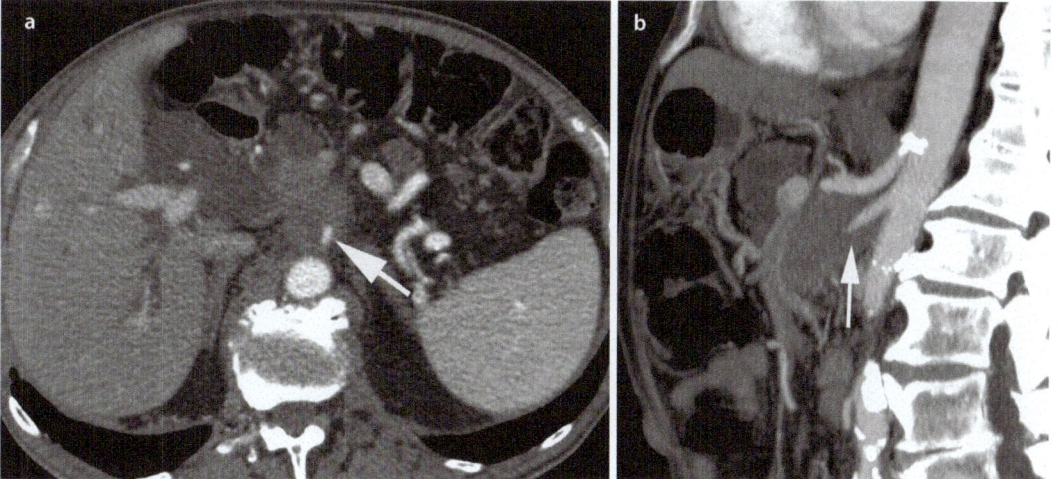

Fig. 6.5 Axial **a** and sagittal **b** CT images show encasement of the SMA (*arrow* in **a** and **b**) and involvement of the retroperitoneal fat, defining this tumor as unresectable

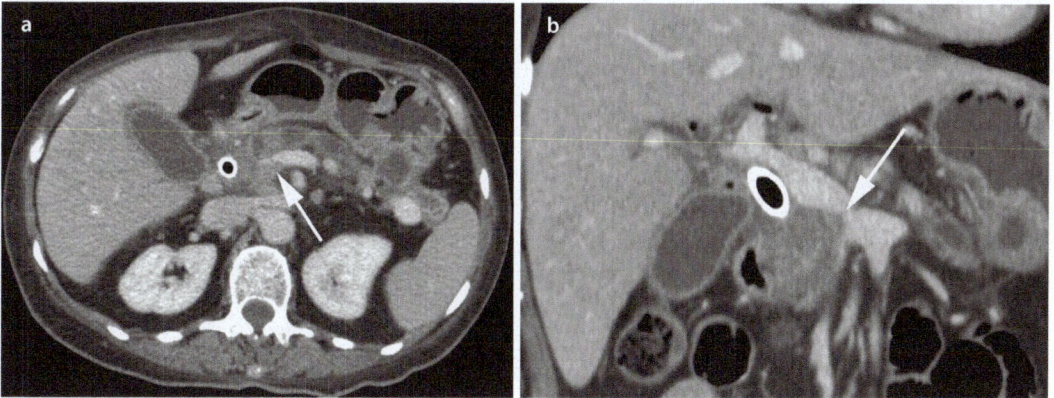

Fig. 6.6 Axial **a** and coronal **b** CT images show a non-reconstructable infiltration of the porto-mesenteric confluence (*arrow* in **a** and **b**)

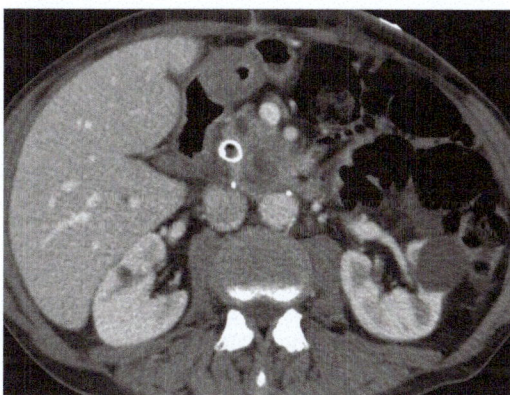

Fig. 6.7 Invasion of the SMA, SMV, and retroperitoneal fat

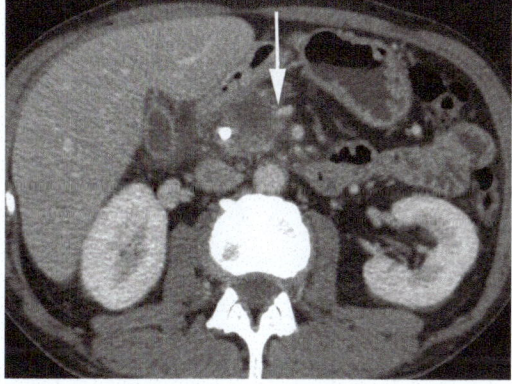

Fig. 6.8 Teardrop mesenteric vein (*arrow*), sign of infiltration of the SMV

6

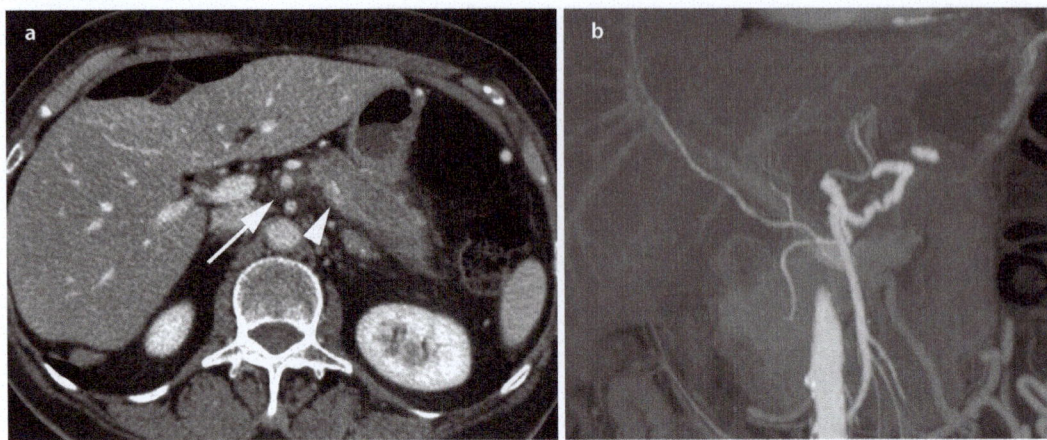

■ **Fig. 6.9** Axial **a** and coronal MIP **b** CT images show infiltration of the splenic vessels (*arrowhead* in **a**) and encasement of the celiac axis >180° (*arrow* in **a**), which makes this tumor unresectable

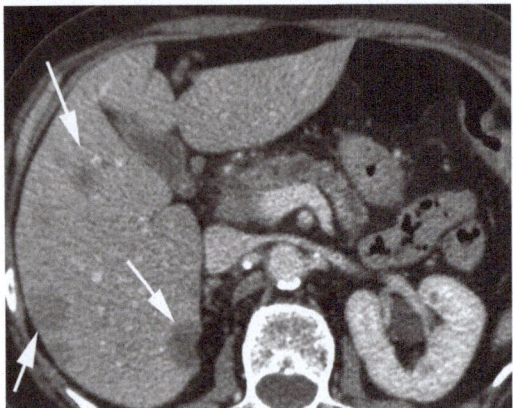

■ **Fig. 6.10** Liver metastases (*arrows*)

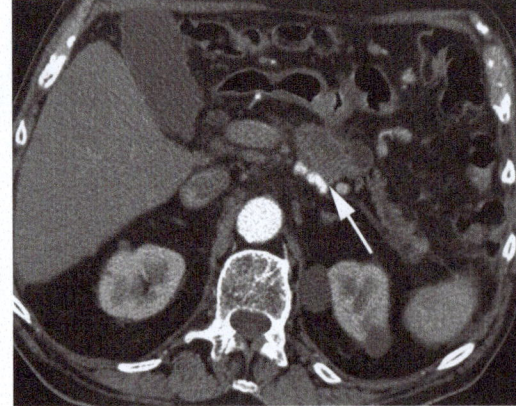

■ **Fig. 6.12** Infiltration of the splenic artery—the tumor is technically resectable; note how the tumor extends dorsally outside the pancreas to reach the artery (*arrow*)

implies more aggressive tumor biology affecting patient prognosis.

6.4 Involvement of Adjacent Organs

Adjacent organs can be involved by direct tumor invasion. The pattern of local extension depends on the site of origin of the tumor.

— Head of pancreas

Invasion of adjacent structures such as the duodenum and the biliary tract constitutes a relatively frequent finding on pancreatico-duodenectomy specimens. Occasionally, tumors originating in the pancreatic head

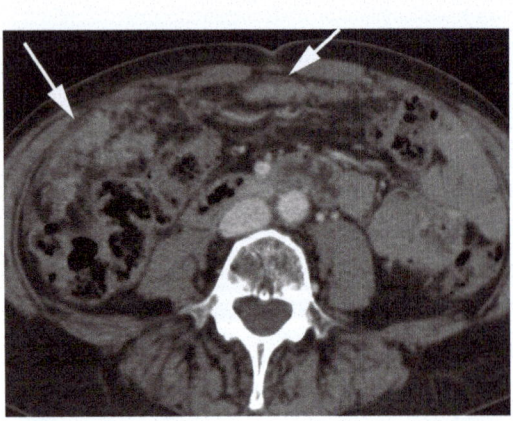

■ **Fig. 6.11** Peritoneal metastases (*arrows*)

It should be therefore noted that—even if a radical resection can be achieved safely from a surgical standpoint—splenic artery involvement

may also involve: colon (right or transverse), transverse mesocolon, small bowel, right kidney and adrenal gland, liver, gallbladder, and diaphragmatic crura.
- Distal pancreas
  Tumors arising in the body or tail of the pancreas can involve the spleen, stomach, colon (transverse or left), transverse mesocolon, small bowel, left kidney and adrenal gland, ligament of Treitz, spine, liver, diaphragmatic crura, and diaphragm.

The ISGPS has provided detailed descriptions of the organs resected during standard pancreaticoduodenectomy and distal pancreatectomy [10]. Every additional resection is considered an extended procedure.

Standard pancreaticoduodenectomy:
- Head of the pancreas and uncinate process
- Duodenum and first segment of jejunum
- Common bile duct and gallbladder
- Lymphadenectomy
- Sometimes pylorus and/or antrum of stomach
- Sometimes elements of the transverse mesocolon exclusive of relevant vasculature (e.g., limited soft tissue contiguous to the tumor but not including the colon itself)

Standard distal pancreatectomy:
- Body and/or tail of the pancreas
- Spleen, including splenic vessels
- Lymphadenectomy
- Sometimes fascia of Gerota
- Sometimes elements of the transverse mesocolon exclusive of relevant vasculature (e.g., limited soft tissue contiguous to the tumor but not including the colon itself)

In the absence of distant metastases, the involvement of adjacent organs does not constitute per se a criterion for non-resectability as far as an extended free-margin tumor resection can be safely performed.

6.5 Lymph Node Involvement

Lymph node metastases have been reported in 60–90% of patients with resected PDAC [11] and lymph node staging is considered one of the strongest prognostic factors after the resection [12].

The precise identification of the specific sequence of lymph node invasion and its correlation with patient survival would be of great value in clinical practice, potentially allowing a better selection of patients undergoing upfront surgery rather than neoadjuvant therapy, and affecting the definition of the optimal extension of lymphadenectomy during resection. The detailed pattern of lymph nodal spread is however difficult to outline, due to the complexity of the anatomical connections between the different lymphatic routes. In addition to this, we must consider the current limitations of even state-of-the-art imaging in the detection of LN metastases. Size-based criteria have been shown to be inadequate for the detection of LN metastases.

Lymph nodes within the pancreatic draining nodal basin are classified into different stations according to the nomenclature proposed by the Japanese Pancreas Society [13]. This nomenclature has reached international acceptance and its use has been also recommended by the latest Consensus Statement of the International Study Group on Pancreatic Surgery [14].

6.5.1 Anatomical Aspects: Tumors of the Pancreatic Head

According to the reports and on the basis of the previous findings of radioisotope and dye injection studies in normal pancreas samples [15–18], two main routes of lymphatic drainage from the pancreatic head were identified (◘ Fig. 6.13):
- The superior part of the head appears to drain to lymph nodes around the celiac axis via the lymph nodes that surround the common hepatic artery.
- The remainder of the head is postulated to drain to lymph nodes around the superior mesenteric artery up to para-aortic lymph nodes.

A more recent study, however, has shown that pancreatic cancer can frequently spread to distant LNs via multiple lymphatic drainage basins without a dominant sentinel location [19].

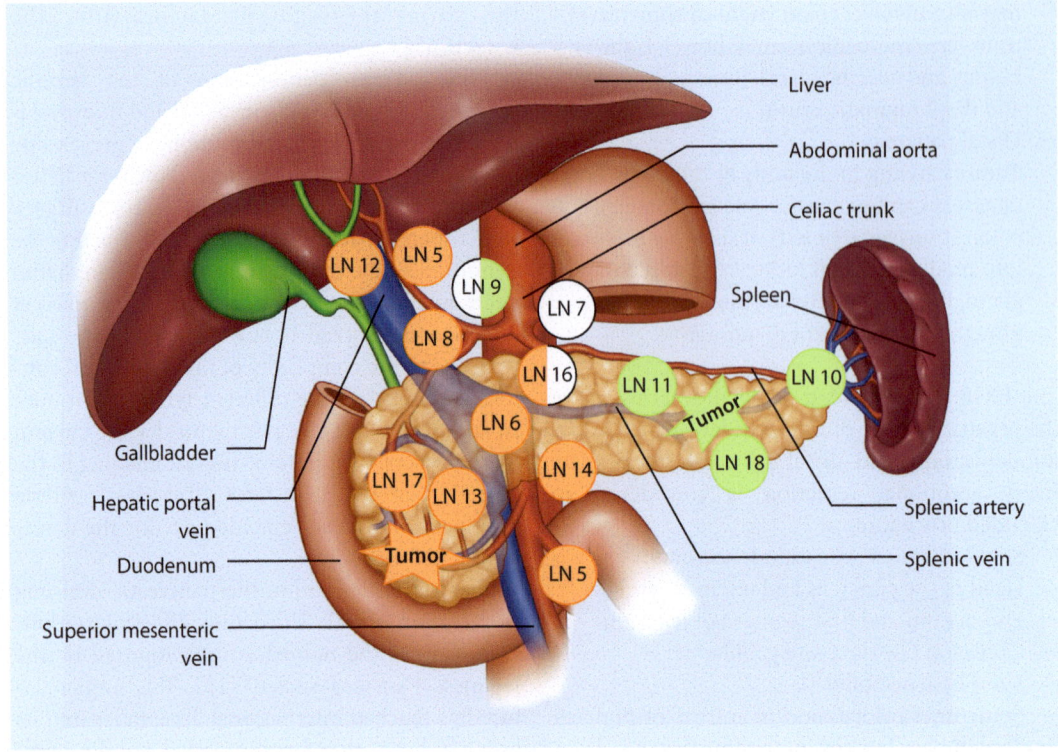

Fig. 6.13 Distribution of lymphatic metastases to lymph node stations from tumors in the pancreatic head (*orange*) and tail (*green*). *LN* Lymph Node Station

6.5.2 The Uncinate Process: A Ventral Enclave in the Dorsal Pancreas

During embryological development, the pancreas arises from the fusion of two independent primordia: the smaller ventral bud forms the caudal part of the pancreatic head and uncinate process, whereas the cephalic part of the pancreatic head, as well as the body and tail, are derived from the larger dorsal bud.

Pancreaticoduodenectomy is generally performed in a similar manner irrespective of the origin of the embryological segment. However, on the basis of their different embryological origins, pancreatic cancers arising in the head and in the uncinate process may actually display peculiar tendencies in local spreading. This fascinating field and its surgical implications have been explored by Japanese authors.

Kitagawa et al. [20] noticed that the lymphatic spread pattern of head PDAC could be attributed to tumor location and speculated that this phenomenon was correlated with the embryological structure of pancreas. The authors showed an exclusive pattern of lymph nodal metastases that was limited to station 8 (along the hepatic artery) and 12 (hepatoduodenal ligament) for tumors almost entirely confined to the dorsal pancreas, and to station 14 (superior mesenteric artery) for tumors almost entirely confined to the ventral pancreas (uncinate process). However, in the case of cancers extending into both domains the lymph node metastases were distributed widely in areas along the superior mesenteric artery, common hepatic artery, and the hepatoduodenal ligament. These results indicate that lymphatic spread of the embryological ventral and dorsal domains of pancreas head carcinomas may be independent of each other even after the fusion of these domains. On this basis, the authors concluded that in order to achieve radical resection during pancreaticoduodenectomy the specific site of lymph node dissection should be guided by the tumor location.

These results were not completely confirmed by the more recent study by Okamura [21], which showed somewhat various and not exclusive lymph nodal metastasis patterns like those of Kitagawa, but confirmed some differences in loco-regional dissemination for pancreatic head tumors arising from the two different primordia. The authors indeed highlighted a significantly higher rate of lymph vessel invasion and of LN station 15 (lymph nodes along the middle colic artery) involvement for tumors arising in the dorsal pancreas, whereas the rate of perineural invasion tended to be higher in tumors arising from the ventral bud.

Comparable findings were reported for patterns of perineural invasion according to the site of origin of the tumor [22], reinforcing the idea that the spread pattern of pancreatic ductal adenocarcinoma of the head and of the uncinate process may differ on the basis of their different embryological development.

Anyway there is currently no evidence supporting the application of different surgical procedures during pancreaticoduodenectomy for tumors arising from the dorsal and ventral pancreas, and further studies are needed to clarify the field.

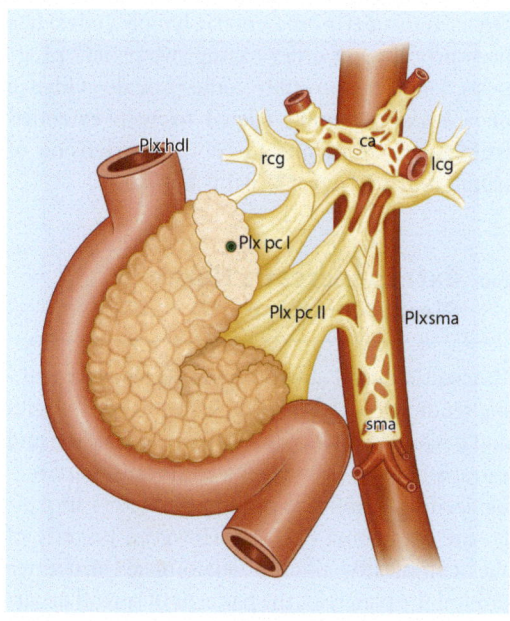

◘ Fig. 6.14 Extrapancreatic nerve plexus

6.5.3 Anatomical Aspects: Tumors of the Distal Pancreas

Based on the anatomical study by Deki and Sato [23], two major lymphatic routes were initially identified in the left half of the pancreas: one follows the splenic blood vessels and the other accompanies the inferior pancreatic artery. By way of these routes, lymphatics from the left half of the pancreas flow into the nodes situated on the left side of the origins of the celiac trunk and superior mesenteric artery (◘ Fig. 6.13).

Early studies [24] suggested a high metastatic rate in lymph nodes along the splenic artery (50%) and the inferior body (35%), around the common hepatic artery (25%) and the para-aortic lymph nodes (20%).

Subsequent studies [25] described quite a different pattern of nodal involvement by distal cancers, with a high metastatic incidence along the splenic artery, superior mesenteric artery, aorta and celiac trunk, and a relatively low incidence on the inferior pancreatic body and around the common hepatic artery.

The important role of stations 11 (splenic artery) and 14 (superior mesenteric artery) as metastatic sites was further confirmed by subsequent studies [26, 27] but a clear route of lymph nodal spreading could not be identified.

Indeed, as pointed out by Fernandez Cruz [28] lymphatic spread of tumors arising in the distal pancreas seems to be less continuous and somewhat "scattered" in comparison with head tumors: through the splenic artery route, these cancers appear to disseminate widely to the retroperitoneum, the para-aortic region, and to other peripancreatic lymph nodes (◘ Fig. 6.14).

6.5.4 Surgical Implications

Despite the recognized prognostic importance of LN variables, the optimal extent of lymphadenectomy during pancreatic resection with radical intent for PDAC is still debated [12].

The performance of extended lymphadenectomy during pancreaticoduodenectomy has not been recommended in clinical practice [14]. However, the interpretation of the current evidence is somewhat hampered by the lack of a common definition of standard lymphadenectomy, preventing comparison of different studies.

As concerns tumors arising in the distal pancreas, studies on lymphadenectomy during left-sided pancreatectomy are scarce. On the basis of the Japanese histopathological studies on the distribution of metastatic lymph nodes, extended lymphadenectomy (including the para-aortic,

6

celiac, and superior mesenteric lymph nodes) has been proposed in order to improve patient prognosis. However, no study could provide evidence on a survival benefit related to such extended lymphadenectomy and the optimal extension of lymph nodal retrieval remains unclear.

6.6 Extrapancreatic Nerve Plexus Invasion

Pancreatic ductal adenocarcinoma shows a striking tendency for perineural invasion both within and beyond the pancreas. Perineural invasion and extrapancreatic nerve plexus infiltration are recognized as significant prognostic factors in pancreatic carcinoma [22, 29]. However, because of the complexity of the anatomical structures around the pancreas, the patterns of spread of carcinoma through the neural stream are difficult to define in details.

Extrapancreatic nerve plexus have been first categorized by Japanese investigators in the 1950s [30]. This classification has been further refined and finally endorsed by the Japanese Pancreas Society, which identifies (◘ Fig. 6.14):

- PL Ph I: Pancreatic head plexus I originates from the right celiac ganglia and enters the superior medial margin of the uncinate process.

- PL Ph II: Pancreatic head plexus II originates from the superior mesenteric plexus and runs as a wide band along the entire length of the medial margin of the uncinate process.
- PL sma: Superior mesenteric arterial plexus.
- PL hdl: Plexus within the hepatoduodenal ligament.
- PL ce: Celiac plexus.
- PL cha: Common hepatic artery plexus.
- PL sp: Splenic plexus.

Head tumors display a more complex spreading pattern, depending on the specific location of the tumor within the pancreatic head. In particular, two main patterns of neural invasion by head PDAC have been identified, in close relationship with the embryological development of the pancreas.

Pathological studies [22] on pancreaticoduodenectomy specimens showed a significant correlation between the tumor location considering the two pancreatic primordia and the site of extrapancreatic nerve plexus infiltration (◘ Fig. 6.15):

- Cancers almost entirely confined to the ventral pancreas extended through the pancreatic head nerve plexus (PL ph1 and PL ph2) to the superior mesenteric nerve plexus (PL sma) (◘ Fig. 6.16).
- Tumors almost entirely confined to the dorsal pancreas tended to involve the neural

◘ **Fig. 6.15** Different routes of perineural invasion for tumors in the pancreatic head (*PH*), uncinate process (*UP*), and body/tail (*PBT*)

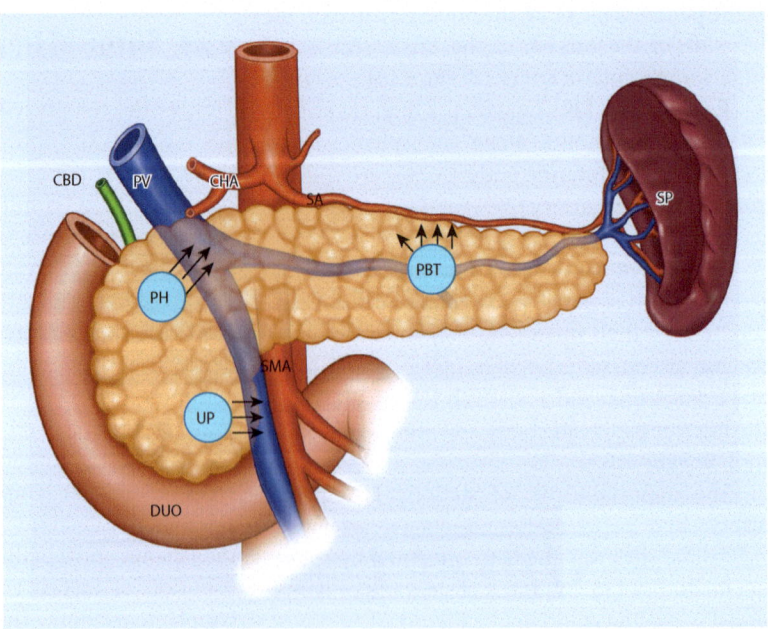

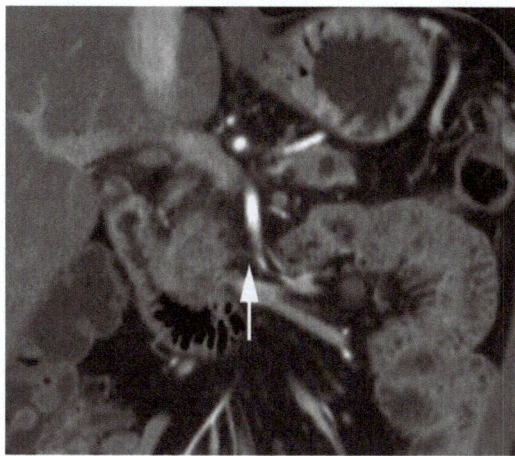

Fig. 6.16 Coronal CT image shows a hypoattenuating tumor in the pancreatic head and spiculations (*arrow*) in the adipose tissue between the pancreatic head and the superior mesenteric artery, consistent with perineural invasion (confirmed at pathology)

plexus around the common hepatic artery (PL cha) and the hepatoduodenal ligament (PL hdl).

In patients with carcinoma of the body and tail of the pancreas, the splenic plexus is the most frequent site of invasion [24]. In addition, a second route of neural invasion has been proposed [31], directly leading to the celiac ganglion via a distinct nerve trunk, which runs independently of blood vessels.

6.6.1 Surgical Implications

While the splenic ganglion is easily removed during distal pancreatectomy, the optimal extent of neural clearance during pancreaticoduodenectomy for pancreatic cancer is still debated. Extended extrapancreatic neural plexus dissection has been advocated, especially by Japanese authors [32], in order to obtain oncologically negative resections and better survival outcomes.

RCTs comparing outcomes of standard and extended lymph node resection failed to show any survival advantages in comparison with standard

resections and were frequently associated with intractable diarrhea [33–37].

Coherently, in the recent ISGPS Guidelines [14] circumferential clearance of the lymph nodes and neural plexus around the superior mesenteric artery has not been recommended, and only tissue at the right side of the superior mesenteric artery has been included in the definition of standard resection.

6.7 Metastatic Spread

The liver is the primary site for hematogenous metastatic spread from the pancreas. The location of the primary tumor influences the distribution of metastases within the liver: tumors located in the body–tail of the pancreas, especially when splenic vein invasion is present, tend to metastasize to the left lobe of the liver more than tumors located in the head of the pancreas [38]. This has been hypothesized to be due to the streamline phenomenon, i.e., the dual blood flow in the portal trunk to the liver: the blood flow from the superior mesenteric vein follows preferentially the right portal trunk to the right lobe of the liver (**Fig. 6.17**). The blood flow from the splenic vein together with the inferior mesenteric vein follows the left side of the portal trunk to the left portal vein and the left lobe of the liver and, because of the smaller caliber of the left portal vein, also enters into the right branch of the portal vein. Therefore, the right lobe of the liver receives the majority of the blood flow, even from the splenic vein.

This streamline phenomenon, already well demonstrated by portal venography studies, can be explained with the shortness of the portal trunk, the smoother angle between the superior mesenteric vein and the right portal vein, and the larger caliber of the right portal vein.

Other less common sites for hematogenous metastases include, in approximate order of frequency, the lungs, adrenals, kidneys, bones, brain, and skin. For dissemination to these sites, no differences have been reported based on the location of the primary tumor.

Fig. 6.17 Distribution of hematogenous metastases to the liver according to the streamline phenomenon theory

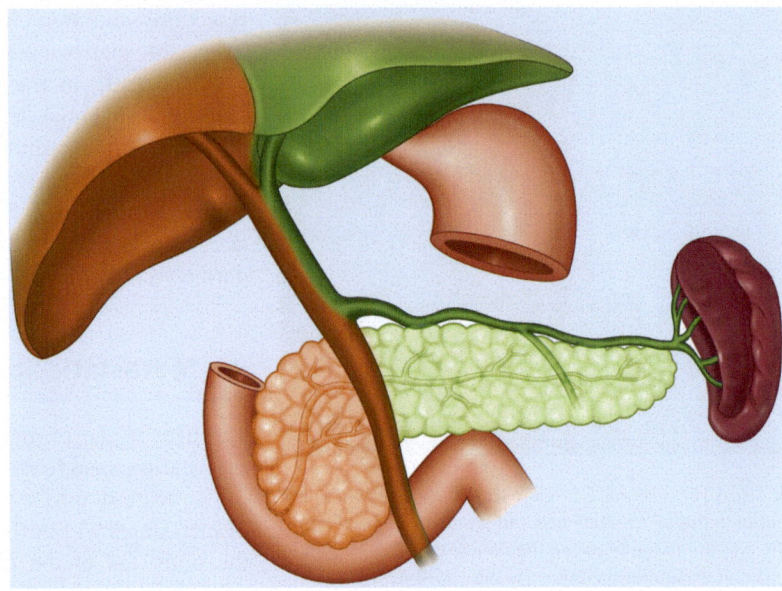

6

References

1. Siegel RL, Miller KD, Jemal A (2015) Cancer statistics, 2015. CA Cancer J Clin 65(1):5–29
2. Pancreatic cancer. http://www.cancer.org/cancer/pancreaticcancer/detailedguide/pancreatic-cancer-key-statistics
3. Raimondi S, Maisonneuve P, Lowenfels AB (2009) Epidemiology of pancreatic cancer: an overview. Nat Rev Gastroenterol Hepatol 6(12):699–708
4. Conroy T, Desseigne F, Ychou M et al (2011) FOLFIRINOX versus gemcitabine for metastatic pancreatic cancer. N Engl J Med 364(19):1817–1825
5. Von Hoff DD, Ervin T, Arena FP et al (2013) Increased survival in pancreatic cancer with nab-paclitaxel plus gemcitabine. N Engl J Med 369(18):1691–1703
6. Kanda M, Fujii T, Sahin TT, Kanzaki A, Nagai S, Yamada S, Sugimoto H, Nomoto S, Takeda S, Kodera Y et al (2010) Invasion of the splenic artery is a crucial prognostic factor in carcinoma of the body and tail of the pancreas. Ann Surg 251(3):483–487
7. Al-Hawary MM, Francis IR, Chari ST, Fishman EK, Hough DM, Lu DS, Macari M, Megibow AJ, Miller FH, Mortele KJ et al (2014) Pancreatic ductal adenocarcinoma radiology reporting template: consensus statement of the Society of Abdominal Radiology and the American Pancreatic Association. Radiology 270(1):248–260
8. Bockhorn M, Uzunoglu FG, Adham M, Imrie C, Milicevic M, Sandberg AA, Asbun HJ, Bassi C, Buchler M, Charnley RM et al (2014) Borderline resectable pancreatic cancer: a consensus statement by the International Study Group of Pancreatic Surgery (ISGPS). Surgery 155(6):977–988
9. Partelli S, Crippa S, Barugola G, Tamburrino D, Capelli P, D'Onofrio M, Pederzoli P, Falconi M (2011) Splenic artery invasion in pancreatic adenocarcinoma of the body and tail: a novel prognostic parameter for patient selection. Ann Surg Oncol 18(13):3608–3614
10. Hartwig W, Vollmer CM, Fingerhut A, Yeo CJ, Neoptolemos JP, Adham M, Andren-Sandberg A, Asbun HJ, Bassi C, Bockhorn M et al (2014) Extended pancreatectomy in pancreatic ductal adenocarcinoma: definition and consensus of the International Study Group for Pancreatic Surgery (ISGPS). Surgery 156(1):1–14
11. Basturk O, Saka B, Balci S, Postlewait LM, Knight J, Goodman M, Kooby D, Sarmiento JM, El-Rayes B, Choi H et al (2015) Substaging of lymph node status in resected pancreatic ductal adenocarcinoma has strong prognostic correlations: proposal for a revised N classification for TNM staging. Ann Surg Oncol 22:S1187–S1195
12. Malleo G, Maggino L, Capelli P, Gulino F, Segattini S, Scarpa A, Bassi C, Butturini G, Salvia R (2015) Reappraisal of nodal staging and study of lymph node station involvement in pancreaticoduodenectomy with the standard international study group of pancreatic surgery definition of lymphadenectomy for cancer. J Am Coll Surg 221(2):367–79.e364
13. Co K (2003) Classification of pancreatic carcinoma. 2nd English ed. Tokyo, Kanehara
14. Tol JA, Gouma DJ, Bassi C, Dervenis C, Montorsi M, Adham M, Andren-Sandberg A, Asbun HJ, Bockhorn M, Buchler MW et al (2014) Definition of a standard lymphadenectomy in surgery for pancreatic ductal adenocarcinoma: a consensus statement by the International Study Group on Pancreatic Surgery (ISGPS). Surgery 156(3):591–600
15. Nagakawa T, Kobayashi H, Ueno K, Ohta T, Kayahara M, Miyazaki I (1994) Clinical study of lymphatic flow to the paraaortic lymph nodes in carcinoma of the head of the pancreas. Cancer 73(4):1155–1162
16. Cubilla AL, Fortner J, Fitzgerald PJ (1978) Lymph node involvement in carcinoma of the head of the pancreas area. Cancer 41(3):880–887
17. Kayahara M, Nagakawa T, Kobayashi H, Mori K, Nakano T, Kadoya N, Ohta T, Ueno K, Miyazaki I (1992)

Lymphatic flow in carcinoma of the head of the pancreas. Cancer 70(8):2061–2066

18. Nakao A, Harada A, Nonami T, Kaneko T, Murakami H, Inoue S, Takeuchi Y, Takagi H (1995) Lymph node metastases in carcinoma of the head of the pancreas region. Br J Surg 82(3):399–402

19. Kanda M, Fujii T, Nagai S, Kodera Y, Kanzaki A, Sahin TT, Hayashi M, Yamada S, Sugimoto H, Nomoto S et al (2011) Pattern of lymph node metastasis spread in pancreatic cancer. Pancreas 40(6):951–955

20. Kitagawa H, Ohta T, Makino I, Tani T, Tajima H, Nakagawara H, Ohnishi I, Takamura H, Kayahara M, Watanabe H et al (2008) Carcinomas of the ventral and dorsal pancreas exhibit different patterns of lymphatic spread. Front Biosci 13:2728–2735

21. Okamura Y, Fujii T, Kanzaki A, Yamada S, Sugimoto H, Nomoto S, Takeda S, Nakao A (2012) Clinicopathologic assessment of pancreatic ductal carcinoma located at the head of the pancreas, in relation to embryonic development. Pancreas 41(4):582–588

22. Makino I, Kitagawa H, Ohta T, Nakagawara H, Tajima H, Ohnishi I, Takamura H, Tani T, Kayahara M (2008) Nerve plexus invasion in pancreatic cancer: spread patterns on histopathologic and embryological analyses. Pancreas 37(4):358–365

23. Deki H, Sato T (1988) An anatomic study of the peripancreatic lymphatics. Surg Radiol Anat 10(2):121–135

24. Kayahara M, Nagakawa T, Futagami F, Kitagawa H, Ohta T, Miyazaki I (1996) Lymphatic flow and neural plexus invasion associated with carcinoma of the body and tail of the pancreas. Cancer 78(12):2485–2491

25. Nakao A, Harada A, Nonami T, Kaneko T, Nomoto S, Koyama H, Kanazumi N, Nakashima N, Takagi H (1997) Lymph node metastasis in carcinoma of the body and tail of the pancreas. Br J Surg 84(8):1090–1092

26. Fujita T, Nakagohri T, Gotohda N, Takahashi S, Konishi M, Kojima M, Kinoshita T (2010) Evaluation of the prognostic factors and significance of lymph node status in invasive ductal carcinoma of the body or tail of the pancreas. Pancreas 39(1):e48–e54

27. Sahin TT, Fujii T, Kanda M, Nagai S, Kodera Y, Kanzaki A, Yamamura K, Sugimoto H, Kasuya H, Nomoto S et al (2011) Prognostic implications of lymph node metastases in carcinoma of the body and tail of the pancreas. Pancreas 40(7):1029–1033

28. Fernandez-Cruz L, Johnson C, Dervenis C (1999) Locoregional dissemination and extended lymphadenectomy in pancreatic cancer. Dig Surg 16(4):313–319

29. Nakao A, Harada A, Nonami T, Kaneko T, Takagi H (1996) Clinical significance of carcinoma invasion of the extrapancreatic nerve plexus in pancreatic cancer. Pancreas 12(4):357–361

30. Yoshioka H, Wakabayashi T (1958) Therapeutic neurotomy on head of pancreas for relief of pain due to chronic pancreatitis; a new technical procedure and its results. AMA Arch Surg 76(4):546–554

31. Yi SQ, Miwa K, Ohta T, Kayahara M, Kitagawa H, Tanaka A, Shimokawa T, Akita K, Tanaka S (2003) Innervation of the pancreas from the perspective of perineural invasion of pancreatic cancer. Pancreas 27(3):225–229

32. Nagakawa T, Kayahara M, Ueno K, Ohta T, Konishi I, Ueda N, Miyazaki I (1992) A clinicopathologic study on neural invasion in cancer of the pancreatic head. Cancer 69(4):930–935

33. Pedrazzoli S, DiCarlo V, Dionigi R, Mosca F, Pederzoli P, Pasquali C, Kloppel G, Dhaene K, Michelassi F (1998) Standard versus extended lymphadenectomy associated with pancreatoduodenectomy in the surgical treatment of adenocarcinoma of the head of the pancreas: a multicenter, prospective, randomized study. Lymphadenectomy Study Group. Ann Surg 228(4):508–517

34. Yeo CJ, Cameron JL, Sohn TA, Coleman J, Sauter PK, Hruban RH, Pitt HA, Lillemoe KD (1999) Pancreaticoduodenectomy with or without extended retroperitoneal lymphadenectomy for periampullary adenocarcinoma: comparison of morbidity and mortality and short-term outcome. Ann Surg 229(5):613–622; discussion 622–4

35. Farnell MB, Pearson RK, Sarr MG, DiMagno EP, Burgart LJ, Dahl TR, Foster N, Sargent DJ (2005) A prospective randomized trial comparing standard pancreatoduodenectomy with pancreatoduodenectomy with extended lymphadenectomy in resectable pancreatic head adenocarcinoma. Surgery 138(4):618–628; discussion 628–30

36. Nimura Y, Nagino M, Takao S, Takada T, Miyazaki K, Kawarada Y, Miyagawa S, Yamaguchi A, Ishiyama S, Takeda Y et al (2012) Standard versus extended lymphadenectomy in radical pancreatoduodenectomy for ductal adenocarcinoma of the head of the pancreas: long-term results of a Japanese multicenter randomized controlled trial. J Hepatobiliary Pancreat Sci 19(3):230–241

37. Jang JY, Kang MJ, Heo JS, Choi SH, Choi DW, Park SJ, Han SS, Yoon DS, Yu HC, Kang KJ et al (2014) A prospective randomized controlled study comparing outcomes of standard resection and extended resection, including dissection of the nerve plexus and various lymph nodes, in patients with pancreatic head cancer. Ann Surg 259(4):656–664

38. Ambrosetti MC, Zamboni GA, Mucelli RP (2016) Distribution of liver metastases based on the site of primary pancreatic carcinoma. Eur Radiol 26:306–310. http://www.ncbi.nlm.nih.gov/pubmed/26017740\t"_blank"

Neuroendocrine Pancreatic Tumors

Marco Miotto, Giovanni Marchegiani, and Giulia Zamboni

© Springer International Publishing AG 2018
D. Regge, G. Zamboni (eds.), *Hepatobiliary and Pancreatic Cancer*,
Cancer Dissemination Pathways, https://doi.org/10.1007/978-3-319-50296-0_7

7

7.1 Overview

7.1.1 Epidemiology

Although often described as rare, the incidence of PNETs has shown a marked increase over the last two decades, thanks to the widespread use of cross-sectional imaging, so that the actual reported incidence for PNETs is 0.32 per 100,000 per year [1]. Autopsy studies searching for small (<1 cm) NETs reported frequencies ranging from 0.8 to 10%.

PNETs are usually solitary and sporadic but in some cases they belong to inherited syndromes, namely: multiple endocrine neoplasia type 1 (MEN1), von Hippel Lindau (VHL), neurofibromatosis type 1 (NF1), and tuberous sclerosis complex (TSC).

7.1.2 Risk Factors

As opposed to pancreatic adenocarcinoma, PNETs have no defined disease-related risk factors.

7.1.3 Pathology

Pancreatic neuroendocrine tumors (PNETs) are a complex and heterogeneous group of rare neoplasms of the pancreas (3%) originating from totipotential stem cells or differentiated mature endocrine cells within the gland.

Pancreatic NETs can be sporadic localized to the head, body, or tail of the gland or they can occur as multiple lesions. MEN-1-associated pancreatic NETs are almost always multifocal and they are usually distributed throughout the pancreatic parenchyma (◻ Fig. 7.1) [2].

Macroscopically, PNETs are usually solitary, solid masses, from 1 to 5 cm in diameter, with rounded borders. The usual PNET is rich in small vessels and has scant fibrotic stroma. It may have unusual features, including cystic aspects, may lead to be misinterpreted as cystic neoplasia; more rarely, they show considerable fibrosis, mimicking ductal adenocarcinoma.

Microscopically, the majority of PNETs are well-differentiated tumors that grow as solid nests or with trabecular patterns, although glandular, acinar, and cribriform features are observed as well.

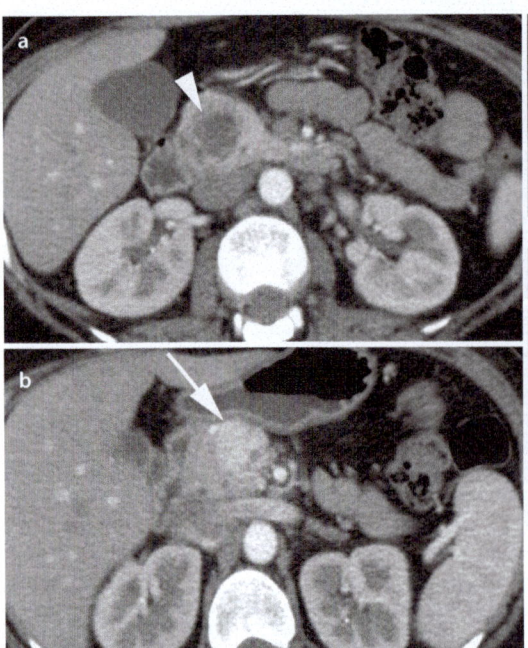
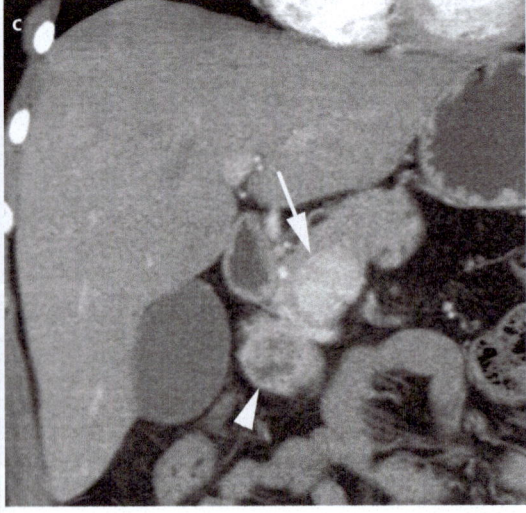

◻ **Fig. 7.1** Axial **a, b** and coronal **c** CT images in a patient affected by MEN-1 show two tumors in the pancreatic head: one in the lower portion is inhomogeneous and hypoattenuating (*arrowhead* in **a**); the second located cranially, is homogeneously hyperattenuating (*arrowhead* in **b**). Both tumors are classified as T3 based on their diameter

7.1.4 Clinical Presentation

Based on the clinical features, PNETs are divided in two categories: functioning (F) or nonfunctioning (NF) neoplasms. F-PNETs present with inappropriate hormone secretion-syndromes and include insulinomas (hypoglycemia), gastrinomas (peptic ulcer, hyperchlorhydria, diarrhea), glucagonomas (hyperglycemic coma, necrolytic migratory erythema), VIPomas (diarrhea), and somatostatinomas (diabetes). NF-PNETs represent the majority (40–80%) of PNETs and mostly present with mass-related symptoms of abdominal pain, nausea, and weight loss or completely asymptomatic and diagnosed incidentally during routine exams (incidentalomas) [3].

7.1.5 Classification and Staging

Since PNETs encompass a wide range of different diseases, it is important to stratify them as precisely as possible, in order to define their biological behavior and orient the most appropriate treatment.

The European Neuroendocrine Tumor Society (ENETS) has recently proposed a prognostic stratification system [4] that takes into account:

- The World Health Organization (WHO) 2010 grading classification, which distinguishes between well-differentiated neuroendocrine tumors (NETs) and poorly differentiated neuroendocrine carcinomas (NECs) of small or large cell type. NETs are then divided according to a grading scheme based on mitotic count or Ki67 index (Table 7.1).
- The Tumor-Node-Metastasis (TNM) staging system, which classifies tumors limited to the

pancreas as T1, T2, or T3 based primarily on dimensions (<2, 2–4, >4 cm). Of note, T3 also includes cases with invasion of the duodenum or bile duct, whereas T4 cases are those with invasion of adjacent organs or large vessels (Table 7.2) (Figs. 7.1, 7.2, 7.3, and 7.4).

7.1.6 Treatment

7.1.6.1 Surgery

In metastatic patients with a reasonable performance status, surgery is recommended in the absence of unresectable lymph node and extra-abdominal metastases, or diffuse unresectable peritoneal carcinomatosis [5]. Potentially curative (R0/R1) surgery should be performed when liver metastases are unilobar (type 1 pattern) in well-differentiated (NET G1–G2) lesions. NEC G3 lesions should not be resected unless they are isolated [6].

Debulking resections (R2), with or without other locoregional or ablative procedures, can be justified as palliative surgical intent in selected patients eligible for aggressive surgery; however, removal of approximately 90% of the tumor volume is recommended.

The resection of the primary tumor, including regional and distal lymph nodes, even in patients with unresectable metastatic liver disease, seems to be related to a better prognosis [7–9] and should be performed prior or synchronous to the treatment of liver metastases.

Liver transplantation may be a therapeutic option in those patients affected by metastatic disease conditioning a hormonal syndrome refractory to all other available treatments, or substitution of liver parenchyma with an increased risk of organ failure. Even if there is a lack of

◻ Table 7.1 World Health Organization 2010 classification of PNETs

Differentiation	Classification	Grade	Mitotic count (per 10 HPF)	Ki-67 index (%)
Well differentiated	NET	G1	<2	≤2
	NET	G2	2–20	3–20
Poorly differentiated	NEC	G3	>20	>20

NET neuroendocrine tumor, *NEC* neuroendocrine carcinoma, *HPF* high power fields

7

◼ Table 7.2 ENETS-TNM 2012 classification	
T-primary tumor	
Tx	Primary tumor cannot be assessed
T0	No evidence of primary tumor
T1	Tumor limited to the pancreas and size <2 cm
T2	Tumor limited to the pancreas and size 2–4 cm
T3	Tumor limited to the pancreas and size >4 cm or invading duodenum or bile duct
T4	Tumor invading adjacent organs (stomach, spleen, colon, adrenal) or wall of large vessel (celiac axis or superior mesenteric artery)
N-regional lymph nodes	
Nx	Regional lymph node cannot be assessed
N0	No regional lymph node metastasis
N1	Regional lymph node metastasis
M-distant metastasis	
Mx	Distant metastasis cannot be assessed
M0	No distant metastasis
M1	Distant metastasis
Stage	
I	T1, N0, M0
IIa	T2, N0, M0
IIb	T3, N0, M0
IIIa	T4, N0, M0
IIIb	Any T, N1, M0
IV	Any T, any N, M1

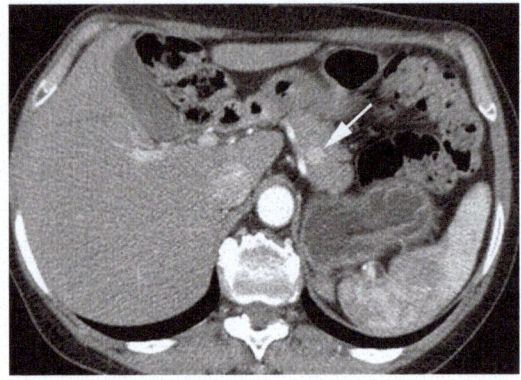

◼ **Fig. 7.2**   Axial arterial phase CT image shows a small homogeneous slightly hypervascular tumor (*arrow*) in the pancreatic tail (T1, G1)

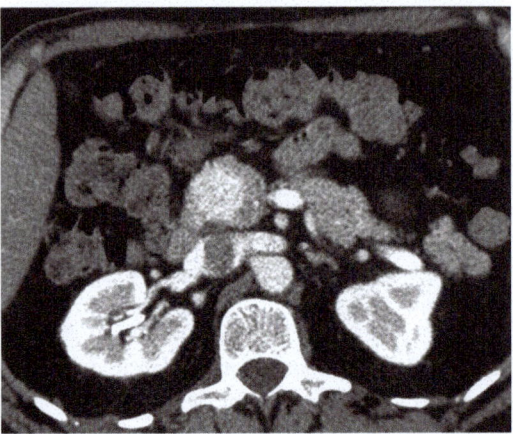

◼ **Fig. 7.3**   Axial arterial phase CT image shows a 3-cm homogeneous hypervascular tumor in the head of the pancreas (T2, G2)

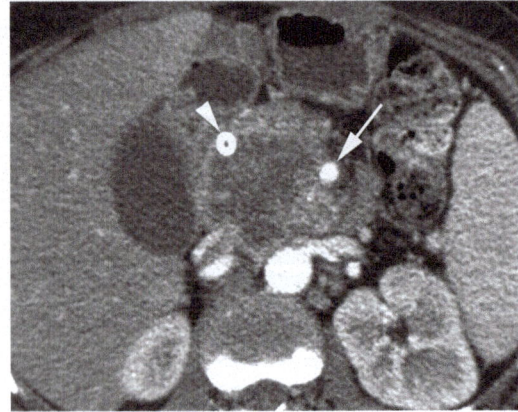

◼ **Fig. 7.4**   Axial arterial phase CT image shows a large inhomogeneous hypodense tumor in the head of the pancreas, which encases the superior mesenteric artery (*arrow*) (T4, G3): a stent is seen in the main bile duct (*arrowhead*)

consensus, the following criteria are minimal requirements for choosing liver transplantation: good performance status, "type 3 pattern" of diffuse G1/G2 disease, absence of unresectable extrahepatic disease [3, 34].

7.1.6.2 Local Ablative and Locoregional Techniques

Radiofrequency ablation (RFA) may be employed for palliation in order to avoid a major surgical procedure and it can also effectively supplement a surgical resection as antitumor treatment and in relieving symptoms in patients with PNET liver metastases (type 2 pattern) less than 5 cm in size [10, 11].

Transcatheter arterial embolization (TAE) or chemoembolization (TACE) may be used to treat liver metastases (G1/G2) in unresectable patients. These procedures are contraindicated in case of complete portal vein thrombosis, hepatic insufficiency, and Whipple procedure [12, 13].

7.1.6.3 Medical Therapy

▪▪ Antiproliferative treatment

Somatostatin analogues (SSA) like Octreotide and Lanreotide are commonly used to treat symptoms associated with hormone hypersecretion in neuroendocrine tumors, and have recently been associated with prolonged progression-free survival among patients with advanced, grade 1 or 2 (Ki-67 < 10%) entero-pancreatic, somatostatin receptor-positive neuroendocrine tumors with prior stable disease, irrespective of the hepatic tumor burden [14, 15].

▪▪ Chemotherapy

Systemic chemotherapy using combinations of streptozotocin and doxorubicin or 5-FU should be considered in patients with advanced unresectable progressive G1–G2 pancreatic NET. Combinations of Etoposide and Cisplatin and more recently Temozolomide are indicated in metastatic NEC G3 [3].

▪▪ Molecular Targeted Therapy

Everolimus and Sunitinib represent novel therapeutic options in patients with surgically non-resectable PNETs after progression following chemotherapy [16–18].

▪▪ PRRT

Peptide Receptor Radionuclide Therapy (PRRT) with radiolabeled somatostatin analogues may be used to treat metastases of G1/G2 NETs and with refractory carcinoid syndrome: the analogues used are ^{90}Y- and/or ^{177}Lu-DOTATOC or -DOTATATE [19, 20].

7.1.7 Prognosis

These tumors are considered less aggressive, when compared with pancreatic adenocarcinoma, on account of their slow growth and also the longer survival observed in patients with advanced disease. Overall the 5-year survival rates range from 38 to 100%, depending on tumor site, stage, and grade.

7.2 Patterns of Local Spread

7.2.1 Introduction

The patterns of diffusion of PNETs such as venous narrowing or occlusion, arterial abutment and arterial encasement are mostly similar to those of ductal adenocarcinoma.

Recent clinical series have started to show some pathological elements that seem to define a distinctive pattern of local spread that includes tumor thrombus and intraductal growth, especially for nonfunctioning PNETS where venous tumor thrombus can extend in the portal, superior mesenteric, and splenic veins (◘ Figs. 7.5 and 7.6). Mechanisms behind this specific pathological and molecular behavior are still unclear [21].

Morphologic (contrast enhanced CT/MRI) and functional (e.g., 68Ga-PET and FDG-PET) imaging are necessary in order to assess the resectability and plan the type of surgical resection [4].

7.3 Vessel Infiltration and Resectability

A tumor is considered resectable when clear anatomical planes can be identified around the celiac axis, hepatic artery, and superior mesenteric

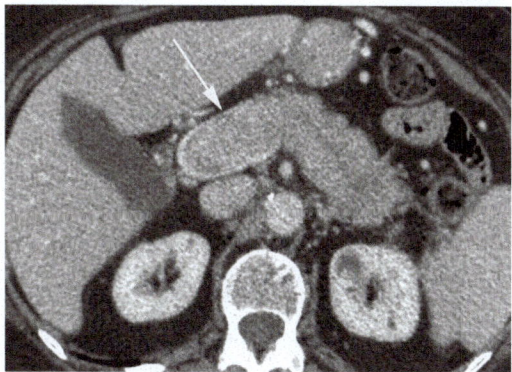

◘ **Fig. 7.5** Venous phase CT image shows a large tumor in the body-tail of the pancreas invading the main trunk of the portal vein with tumor thrombus (*arrow*)

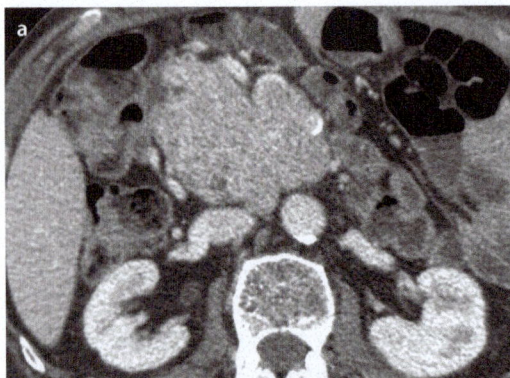

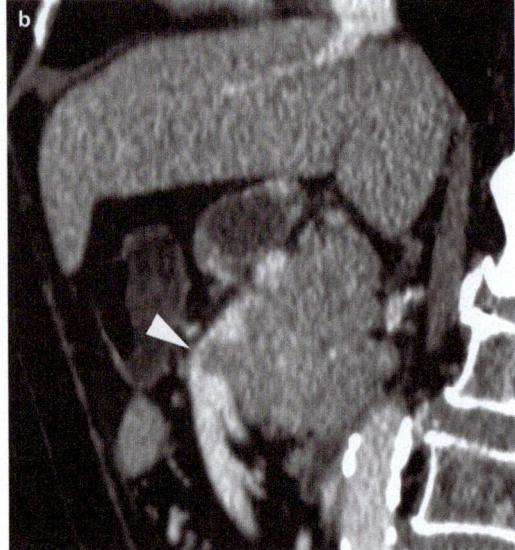

Fig. 7.6 Axial **a** and coronal **b** CT images show a large inhomogeneous tumor in the pancreatic head and body that encases the SMA and invades the SMV (*arrowhead* in **b**)

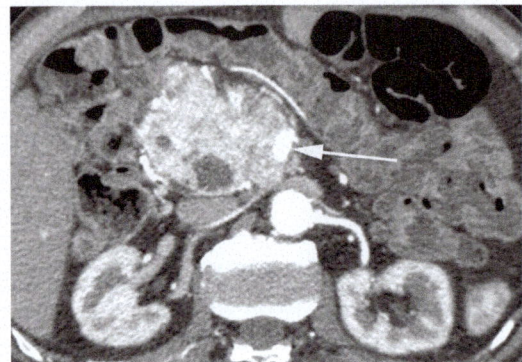

Fig. 7.7 Arterial phase CT shows a large inhomogeneous tumor in the pancreatic head that encases the SMA (*arrow*)

artery, and there is no radiologic evidence of superior mesenteric vein or portal vein distortion. "Borderline-resectable" neoplasm definition and patterns of vessel are not peculiar, and follow those already described for PDAC in ▶ Chap. 5.

The resectability of NF pancreatic NETs should be assessed preoperatively. Surgical resection is contraindicated under the following conditions: (1) circumferential invasion of portal vein system with portal cavernoma (tumor thrombus excluded), and (2) circumferential invasion of superior mesenteric artery (● Figs. 7.6 and 7.7). The presence of celiac trunk invasion is not an absolute contraindication for distal pancreatectomy [4].

Surgical resection should be considered also in cases with vascular abutment or invasion, in ter-

tiary care centers [22]. Norton et al., in their series, described a good oncological outcome and acceptable postoperative complication rate in patients who underwent aggressive surgery. Extended vascular (venous and arterial) resections and liver resection for vascular invasion and simple pattern liver metastatic disease, respectively, could be a considerable therapeutic option [23].

The presence of portal vein thrombi in patients with PanNETs is not rare and does not represent a contraindication to surgery. A recent study has described the removal of the thrombus as a safe and feasible procedure in highly selected patients and following specific precautions: (a) the tumor thrombus must be mobile as an appendage from the primitive tumor (i.e., without vessel encasement); (b) if needed, multivisceral and/or additional vessels resections should be performed before thrombectomy, and (c) a multimodal therapeutic strategy should be considered before performing surgery (e.g., citoreductive treatment) [24].

7.4 Involvement of Adjacent Organs

Direct tumor invasion can occur for PNETs, depending on the primary tumor localization (head or distal pancreas), as described for pancreatic ductal adenocarcinoma (see ▶ Chap. 5) (● Figs. 7.8 and 7.9). When surgery is warranted, distal or total pancreatectomy with multivisceral resection (partial/subtotal gastrectomy, nephrectomy, left colectomy) can be feasible.

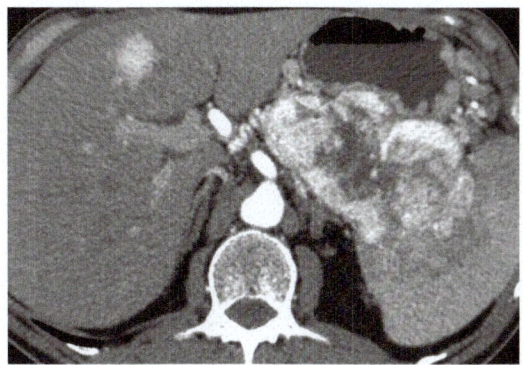

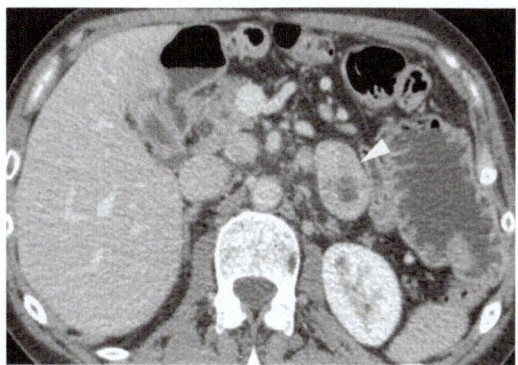

◻ Fig. 7.8   A large inhomogeneous tumor in the body-tail of the pancreas that encases the splenic vessels and invades the splenic parenchyma; a hypervascular liver metastasis is also observed

◻ Fig. 7.10   CT shows several enlarged lymphnodes in the retroperitoneum. The largest (*arrowhead*) has inhomogeneous enhancement and a fluid portion compatible with necrosis

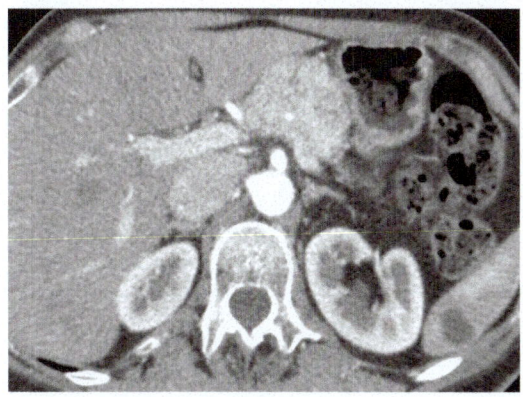

◻ Fig. 7.9   A large hypervascular tumor in the body-tail of the pancreas abutting the lesser gastric curvature, without a clear resection plane

7.5   Lymphnode Involvement

The prevalence of reported lymph node metastases ranges from about 40% in NF-PNETs to up to 80% in gastrinomas [25]. Although the lymphatic spread scheme can be similar to PDAC, small G1 nonfunctioning neoplasms are associated with a lower risk of positive lymph nodes and related to a better prognosis.

Recent studies have reported that the presences of lymph nodes, and their number in some of these studies, have important prognostic value in PNET patients. These results support the recommendation that systematic removal of lymph nodes in the peritumoral area should be routinely performed in any PNET resection. When lymph nodes are involved, a positive nodal status, the number of involved lymph node, as well as the ratio of positive lymph nodes and total retrieved lymph nodes are important independent predictors of recurrence after surgery [22].

Although several studies have demonstrated that proper staging for many types of gastrointestinal cancers requires the evaluation of a minimum number of lymph nodes, no threshold has been established for PNETs [26].

Once again, we must remember the current limitations of even state-of-the-art imaging in the detection of LN metastases, and the inadequacy of size-based criteria (◻ Fig. 7.10).

7.6   Extrapancreatic Nerve Plexus Invasion

Due to the lack of studies, mechanisms behind neural invasion by the PNETs are not clear.

Neural invasion is observed in a high number of PNETs irrespective of functional activity, hormonal subtype, or histology. It is more frequently found in high grade PNETs and in tumors that display entrapments of islets and a higher mitotic activity, reflecting a more aggressive nature [27]. Similarly to what described for PDAC, the expression of epidermal growth factor receptor (EGFR) and nerve growth factor (NGF) appears to be associated with a higher rate of perineural invasion. This invasion, however, is usually microscopical and confined within tumor boundaries: once the tumor is resected, therefore, the perineural and epineural tumor propagations

7

appear to be removed together with the tumoral mass without having spread beyond the tumor borders [27].

7.7 Metastatic Spread

PNETs represent an important clinical issue because of their high percentage of metastatization. Liver metastases, especially from a nonfunctioning primitive tumor [4], are found in 40–45% up to 73% of patients at the time of initial diagnosis, and the presence of metastases represents the most crucial prognostic factor [28].

In international databases, the median survival in distant metastatic disease was 33 months in patients with G1-G2 NETs, but only 5 months in patients with poorly differentiated carcinomas/NEC G3, and 5-year survival rates around 40–60% [29, 30].

7.7.1 Liver Metastases

7.7.1.1 Pattern of Metastases

Macroscopically, three different patterns of liver infiltration by metastases have been described [31, 32] (◘ Table 7.3):

1. Liver metastases confined to one liver lobe or limited to two adjacent segments. This "simple pattern" can be found in 20–25% of the cases (◘ Fig. 7.11).
2. Liver metastases with a "complex pattern," i.e., with one lobe primarily affected but with smaller contralateral lesions occurring in 10–15% of the cases (◘ Fig. 7.12).
3. Diffuse, multifocal liver metastases are found in 60–70% of the cases (◘ Fig. 7.13).

◘ **Table 7.3** Pattern of metastatic spread to the liver

Pattern	Diffusion
Type 1—simple	One lobe or two adjacent segments
Type 2—complex	One lobe and smaller satellites
Type 3—diffuse	Multifocal lesions to all the liver

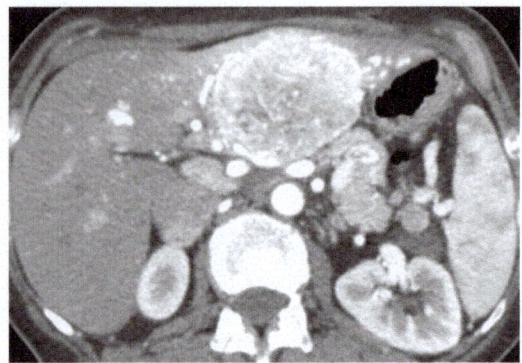

◘ **Fig. 7.11** CT shows one single large metastasis in the left liver lobe (simple pattern, type 1)

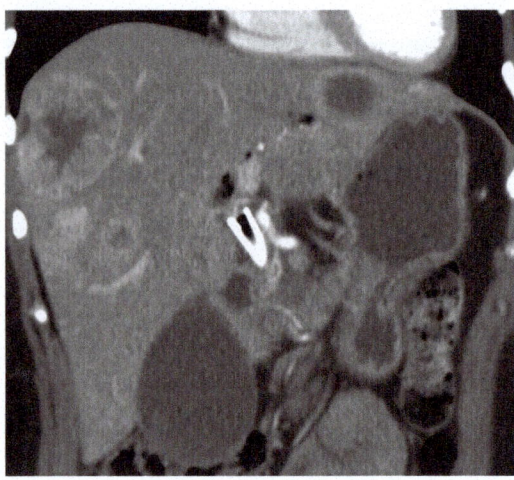

◘ **Fig. 7.12** CT shows that the right liver lobe is predominantly affected by metastases, while one single lesion is seen in the left lobe (complex pattern, type 2)

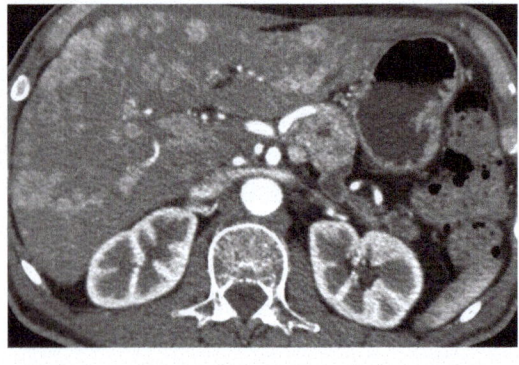

◘ **Fig. 7.13** CT shows innumerable liver metastases distributed to all segment (diffuse pattern, type 3)

7.7.1.2 Predisposing/Predictive Factors of Metastasis

- **Grading**: Ki-67 labeling index reflects the biological behavior and is strongly correlated with the malignant potential of the primitive disease. European and SEER (the largest US epidemiological database) series confirmed this aspect: 50% of patients with poorly differentiated neuroendocrine carcinomas (NEC G3) had distant metastases at initial diagnosis, whereas only 21 and 30% of patients with well-differentiated and moderately differentiated neuroendocrine tumors (NET G1 and G2) showed distant metastases at initial diagnosis, respectively [33].
- **T-Stage**: In NF-PNETs a primitive tumor size >2 cm increases the risk of malignancy compared to T ≤ 2 cm. It must be underlined that even in this last group of smaller tumors, in some series 10% up to 19% of patients presented metastatic lymph nodes at final histological exam [34, 35].
- **Functionality** is associated with metastatic disease depending on the tumor cell type:
  - *Insulinoma*: Mostly benign tumor that metastasizes in <10% of cases [36].
  - *Gastrinoma*: Metastases are very frequent and occur first in regional lymph nodes and in the liver (70–80% at diagnosis) and later in the skeleton (12%). Metastatic Zollinger-Ellison Syndrome (ZES) indicates a bad prognosis disease with a 10-year overall survival (OS) of 30% [37].
  - *VIPoma*: 56% and 64% rate of metastases and malignancy, respectively, as described in large series, with a 5-year survival rate of 60% [38].
  - *Glucagonoma*: Almost 60% of patients have already metastases at the time of diagnosis [39].
  - *Somatostatinoma*: 80% are malignant, of large size, and present with liver metastases [40].

7.7.2 PNETs Metastatic to Other Organs

Occasionally liver metastases from PNETs may be associated with extrahepatic metastases including peritoneal cavity (■ Fig. 7.14), lung, bone, and other metastatic disease sites (e.g., brain, heart, ovaries) with still unclear mechanisms [30, 32, 41–43].

7.7.2.1 Bone Metastases

In a recent series bone metastases occurred in 8% of pancreatic NETs (12 out of 153) [44]. They are often asymptomatic and found during staging exams. The most common symptoms are pain, pathological fractures, and hypercalcemia-related symptoms [29].

7.7.2.2 Lung Metastases

According to the literature, 4–15% of GEP-NETs present with lung metastases in the advanced stage of the disease. Although usually asymptomatic, patients may present with cough, hemoptysis, and pneumonia, a classical triad caused by luminal obstruction and tumor ulceration [29].

7.7.2.3 Cardiac Metastases

The incidence in patients with NETs is <1%. They occur late in the course of the disease and are observed irrespective of the presence of carcinoid valvular disease. However, they are almost always associated with other metastases and liver involvement. The occurrence of myocardial metastases has been described more often in patients with functioning tumors than in those with nonfunctioning tumors [30–32, 43].

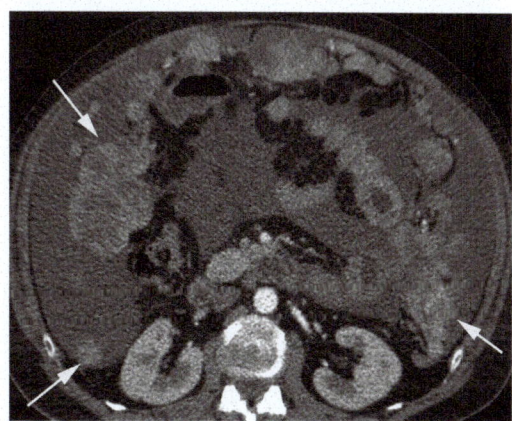

■ **Fig. 7.14** Multiple peritoneal nodules compatible with carcinomatosis (*arrows*)

7.7.2.4 Ovarian Metastases

They represent approximately 2% of all NETs metastases, but are extremely rare with pancreatic primary tumors and are more common with ileum and appendix carcinoid tumors. They are usually bilateral in contrast to primary ovarian lesions, which are usually unilateral, and this constitutes a significant point in terms of differential diagnosis [30].

References

1. Yao JC, Hassan M, Phan A et al (2008) One hundred years after "carcinoid": epidemiology of and prognostic factors for neuroendocrine tumors in 35,825 cases in the United States. J Clin Oncol 26:3063–3072

2. Triponez F, Dosseh D, Goudet P et al (2006) Epidemiology data on 108 MEN 1 patients from the GTE with isolated nonfunctioning tumors of the pancreas. Ann Surg 243(2):265–272. https://doi.org/10.1097/01.sla.0000197715.96762.68

3. Pederzoli P, Bassi C (eds) (2013) Uncommon pancreatic neoplasms, updates in surgery©. Springer, Milano

4. Falconi M, Bartsch DK, Eriksson B et al (2012) ENETS Consensus Guidelines for the management of patients with digestive neuroendocrine neoplasms of the digestive system: well-differentiated pancreatic nonfunctioning tumors. Neuroendocrinology 95:120–134. https://doi.org/10.1159/000335587

5. Frilling A, Sotiropoulos GC, Li J, Kornasiewicz O, Plöckinger U (2010) Multimodal management of neuroendocrine liver metastases. HPB 12(6):361–379. https://doi.org/10.1111/j.1477-2574.2010.00175.x

6. Cho CS, Labow DM, Tang L et al (2008) Histologic grade is correlated with outcome after resection of hepatic neuroendocrine neoplasms. Cancer 113:126–134

7. Capurso G, Bettini R, Rinzivillo M, Boninsegna L, Delle Fave G, Falconi M (2011) Role of resection of the primary pancreatic neuroendocrine tumour only in patients with unresectable metastatic liver disease: a systematic review. Neuroendocrinology 93(4):223–229. https://doi.org/10.1159/000324770

8. Bertani E, Fazio N, Botteri E et al (2014) Resection of the primary pancreatic neuroendocrine tumor in patients with unresectable liver metastases: possible indications for a multimodal approach. Surgery 155(4):607–614. https://doi.org/10.1016/j.surg.2013.12.024

9. Hüttner FJ, Schneider L, Tarantino I et al (2015) Palliative resection of the primary tumor in 442 metastasized neuroendocrine tumors of the pancreas: a population-based, propensity score-matched survival analysis. Langenbecks Arch Surg 400:1–9. https://doi.org/10.1007/s00423-015-1323-x

10. Eriksson J, Stålberg P, Nilsson A, Krause J, Lundberg C, Skogseid B et al (2008) Surgery and radiofrequency ablation for treatment of liver metastases from midgut and foregut carcinoids and endocrine pancreatic tumors. World J Surg 32:930–938

11. Evard S, Becouarn Y, Fonck M, Brunet R, Mathoulin-Pelissier S, Picot V (2004) Surgical treatment of liver metastases by radiofrequency ablation, resection, or in combination. Eur J Surg Oncol 30:399–406

12. Roche A, Girish BV, de Baere T, Baudin E, Boige V, Elias D et al (2003) Trans-catheter arterial chemoembolization as first-line treatment for hepatic metastases from endocrine tumors. Eur Radiol 13:136–140

13. Vogl TJ, Naguib NN, Zangos S, Eichler K, Hedayati A, Nour-Eldin NE (2009) Liver metastases of neuroendocrine carcinomas: interventional treatment via transarterial embolization, chemoembolization and thermal ablation. Eur J Radiol 72:517–528

14. Rinke A, Müller H-H, Schade-Brittinger C et al (2009) Placebo-controlled, double-blind, prospective, randomized study on the effect of octreotide LAR in the control of tumor growth in patients with metastatic neuroendocrine midgut tumors: a report from the PROMID Study Group. J Clin Oncol 27(28):4656–4663. https://doi.org/10.1200/JCO.2009.22.8510

15. Caplin ME, Pavel M, Ćwikła JB et al (2014) Lanreotide in metastatic enteropancreatic neuroendocrine tumors. N Engl J Med 371(3):224–233. https://doi.org/10.1056/NEJMoa1316158

16. Yao JC et al (2011) Everolimus for advanced pancreatic neuroendocrine tumors. N Engl J Med 364:514–523

17. Raymond E, Dahan L, Raoul J-L et al (2011) Sunitinib malate for the treatment of pancreatic neuroendocrine tumors. N Engl J Med 364(6):501–513. https://doi.org/10.1056/NEJMoa1003825

18. Pavel ME, Hainsworth JD, Baudin E, Peeters M, Hörsch D, Winkler RE, Klimovsky J, Lebwohl D, Jehl V, Wolin EM, Öberg K, Van Cutsem E, Yao JC, RADIANT-2 Study Group (2011) Everolimus plus octreotide long-acting repeatable for the treatment of advanced neuroendocrine tumours associated with carcinoid syndrome (RADIANT-2): a randomised, placebo-controlled, phase 3 study. Lancet 378(9808):2005–2012. https://doi.org/10.1016/S0140-6736(11)61742-X

19. Kwekkeboom DJ, de Herder WW, Kam BL et al (2008) Treatment with the radiolabeled somatostatin analog [^{177}Lu-DOTA^0,Tyr^3]octreotate: toxicity, efficacy, and survival. J Clin Oncol 26:2124–2130

20. Bushnell DL Jr, O'Dorisio TM, O'Dorisio MS, Menda Y, Hicks RJ, Van Cutsem E et al (2010) ^{90}Y-edotreotide for metastatic carcinoid refractory to octreotide. J Clin Oncol 28:1652–1659

21. Balachandran A, Tamm EP, Bhosale PR et al (2012) Venous tumor thrombus in nonfunctional pancreatic neuroendocrine tumors. Am J Roentgenol 199(3):602–608. https://doi.org/10.2214/AJR.11.7058

22. Falconi M, Eriksson B, Kaltsas G et al (2016) ENETS consensus guidelines update for the management of patients with functional pancreatic neuroendocrine tumors and non-functional pancreatic neuroendocrine tumors. Neuroendocrinology 103(2):153–171. https://doi.org/10.1159/000443171

23. Norton JA (2011) Pancreatic endocrine tumors with major vascular abutment, involvement, or encasement and indication for resection. Arch Surg 146(6):724–732. https://doi.org/10.1001/archsurg.2011.129

24. Prakash L, Lee JE, Yao J et al (2015) Role and operative technique of portal venous tumor thrombectomy in patients with pancreatic neuroendocrine tumors. J Gastrointest Surg 19(11):2011–2018

25. Giovinazzo F, Butturini G, Monsellato D, Malleo G, Marchegiani G, Bassi C (2013) Lymph nodes metastasis and recurrences justify an aggressive treatment of gastrinoma. Updat Surg 65(1):19–24. https://doi.org/10.1007/s13304-013-0201-8

26. Parekh JR, Wang SC, Bergsland EK et al (2012) Lymph node sampling rates and predictors of nodal metastasis in pancreatic neuroendocrine tumor resections: the UCSF experience with 149 patients. Pancreas 41(6):840–844. https://doi.org/10.1097/MPA.0b013e31823cdaa0

27. Bergmann F, Ceyhan GO, Rieker RJ et al (2009) Fundamental differences in the neural invasion behavior of pancreatic endocrine tumors: relevance for local recurrence rates? Hum Pathol 40(1):50–57. https://doi.org/10.1016/j.humpath.2008.06.021

28. Pape UF, Berndt U, Müller-Nordhorn J, Böhmig M, Roll S, Koch M, Willich SN, Wiedenmann B (2008) Prognostic factors of long-term outcome in gastroenteropancreatic neuroendocrine tumours. Endocr Relat Cancer 15:1083–1097

29. Ekeblad S, Skogseid B, Dunder K, Öberg K, Eriksson B (2008) Prognostic factors and survival in 324 patients with pancreatic endocrine tumor treated at a single institution. Clin Cancer Res 14(23):7798–7803. https://doi.org/10.1158/1078-0432.CCR-08-0734

30. Birnbaum DJ, Turrini O, Ewald J et al (2014) Pancreatic neuroendocrine tumor: a multivariate analysis of factors influencing survival. Eur J Surg Oncol 40(11):1564–1571. https://doi.org/10.1016/j.ejso.2014.06.004

31. Steinmüller T, Kianmanesh R, Falconi M, Scarpa A, Taal B, Kwekkeboom DJ et al (2008) Consensus guidelines for the management of patients with liver metastases from digestive (neuro) endocrine tumors: foregut, midgut, hindgut, and unknown primary. Neuroendocrinology 87:47–62

32. Pavel M, Grossman A, Arnold R et al (2010) ENETS consensus guidelines for the management of brain, cardiac and ovarian metastases from neuroendocrine tumors. Neuroendocrinology 91:326–332. https://doi.org/10.1159/000287277

33. Cherenfant J, Talamonti MS, Hall CR et al (2014) Comparison of tumor markers for predicting outcomes after resection of nonfunctioning pancreatic neuroendocrine tumors. Surgery 156(6):1504–10; discussion 1510–1. https://doi.org/10.1016/j.surg.2014.08.043

34. Bettini R, Partelli S, Boninsegna L et al (2011) Tumor size correlates with malignancy in nonfunctioning pancreatic endocrine tumor. Surgery 150(1):75–82. https://doi.org/10.1016/j.surg.2011.02.022

35. Crippa S, Partelli S, Zamboni G, Scarpa A, Tamburrino D, Bassi C et al (2014) Incidental diagnosis as prognostic factor in different tumor stages of nonfunctioning pancreatic endocrine tumors. Surgery 155(1):145–153. https://doi.org/10.1016/j.surg.2013.08.002

36. Davì MV, Falconi M (2009) Pancreas: insulinoma—new insights into an old disease. Nat Rev Endocrinol 5:300–302

37. Weber HC, Venzon DJ, Lin JT et al (1995) Determinants of metastatic rate and survival in patients with Zollinger-Ellison syndrome: a prospective long-term study. Gastroenterology 108:1637–1649

38. Soga J, Yakuwa Y (1998) Vipoma/diarrheogenic syndrome: a statistical evaluation of 241 reported cases. J Exp Clin Cancer Res 17:389–400

39. Hellman P, Andersson M, Rastad J et al (2000) Surgical strategy for large or malignant endocrine pancreatic tumors. World J Surg 24:1353–1360

40. Krejs GJ, Orci L, Conlon JM et al (1979) Somatostatinoma syndrome. Biochemical, morphologic and clinical features. N Engl J Med 301:285–292

41. Kos-Kudla B, O'Toole D, Falconi M, Gross D, Klöppel G, Sundin A et al (2010) ENETS consensus guidelines for the management of bone and lung metastases from neuroendocrine tumors. Neuroendocrinology 91:341–350

42. Kianmanesh R, Ruszniewski P, Rindi G, Kwekkeboom D, Pape UF, Kulke M et al (2010) ENETS consensus guidelines for the management of peritoneal carcinomatosis from neuroendocrine tumors. Neuroendocrinology 91:333–340

43. Penz M, Kurtaran A, Vorbeck F, Oberhuber G, Raderer M (2000) Case 2: myocardial metastases from a carcinoid tumor. J Clin Oncol 18(7):1596–1597

44. Van Loon K, Zhang L, Keiser J et al (2015) Bone metastases and skeletal-related events from neuroendocrine tumors. Endocr Connect 4(1):9–17. https://doi.org/10.1530/EC-14-0119

Mucinous Carcinoma and IPMN

Maria Chiara Ambrosetti, Matilde Bacchion, Alex Borin,
and Roberto Pozzi Mucelli

© Springer International Publishing AG 2018
D. Regge, G. Zamboni (eds.), *Hepatobiliary and Pancreatic Cancer*,
Cancer Dissemination Pathways, https://doi.org/10.1007/978-3-319-50296-0_8

Mucin-producing tumors of the pancreas represent a group of premalignant or malignant neoplasms forming multilocular cysts and lined by tall, columnar mucinous epithelium. These tumors are broadly divided into mucinous cystic neoplasms (MCN) and intraductal papillary mucinous neoplasms (IPMN) which have different biologic behavior and pathologic features, including prevalence of invasive cancer, recurrence rate after radical resection, and presence of multifocal lesions. For these reasons a deep knowledge of the imaging features and preferential pathways of local or distal tumor spread focusing on parenchymal, vascular, nodal, perineural, and peritoneal dissemination may improve the radiologist's confidence when assessing these diseases.

Mucin-producing tumors of the pancreas represent a group of premalignant or malignant neoplasms forming multilocular cysts and lined by tall, columnar mucinous epithelium. These tumors are broadly divided into mucinous cystic neoplasms (MCN) and intraductal papillary mucinous neoplasms (IPMN) [1].

8.1 Mucinous Adenocarcinoma

Until 1978 there was no distinction between serous and mucinous cystadenomas of the pancreas [2]. A few years later, in 1982, Ohashi et al. published the first description of what now we refer to as IPMNs [3]. In 1996 first, and then in 2000 the World Health Organization (WHO) definitively differentiated these two entities and defined the presence of ovarian stroma as peculiar to mucinous cystic neoplasms of the pancreas (MCN). Afterwards many international consensus conferences, up to the Sendai classification, have proposed guidelines for the diagnosis and management of MCN.

8.1.1 Epidemiology

Mucinous cystic neoplasms represent approximately 10% of pancreatic cysts and 1% of pancreatic neoplasms. They are found almost exclusively in women (>95% of cases) in their 4th to 6th decades of life. However, there is a spectrum and cases have been described in women ranging from 20 to 95 years of age [4]. Complete surgical excision of this group of pancreatic neoplasms usually results in an excellent prognosis (94% 5-year survival) without any additional therapy being indicated. Clinical follow-up is however suggested, often for a prolonged period, as the tumors are slow-growing and may recur after several years. The 5-year disease-specific survival for noninvasive MCNs is 100%, and for those with invasive cancer 57%. Patients with malignant tumors are reported to be 5.5 years older than those with adenoma and borderline neoplasms, and patients with invasive carcinoma were 11 years older than those with noninvasive MCNs. Whether the benign-appearing epithelium transforms into malignant epithelium in a teleologic development of the tumor or whether the malignant epithelium "matures" into a benign-appearing epithelium is unknown. For these reasons, none of the tumors within the MCN category should ever be regarded as truly benign, but instead as low-grade malignant tumors.

8.1.2 Pathology

Mucinous cystic neoplasms (MCNs) usually are large, septated, thick-walled mucinous cysts that lack communication with the ductal system, and occur almost exclusively in the body and tail of pancreas.

The pathogenesis of mucinous cystic neoplasm of the pancreas is uncertain. However, this lesion shares both clinical and pathologic characteristics with biliary and ovarian mucinous tumors. It has been speculated that the embryologic origins of these lesions may be related to germ cell migration in early fetal life during the first 8 weeks of gestation. Each of these tumors is characterized by two distinct histologic components: an inner epithelial layer composed of tall mucin-secreting cells, and a dense cellular ovarian-type stroma. The latter was first described by Compagno and Oertel in 1978, who made a clear distinction between these neoplasms and serous cystic tumors. However, the presence of ovarian stroma was not considered a specific diagnostic criterion for MCNs until a recent consensus conference held in Sendai, Japan, where the International Association of Pancreatology proposed guidelines requiring the presence of ovarian stroma to establish the diagnosis of MCNs [5]. The entire tumor is usually encapsulated by an outer layer of fibrous connective tissue.

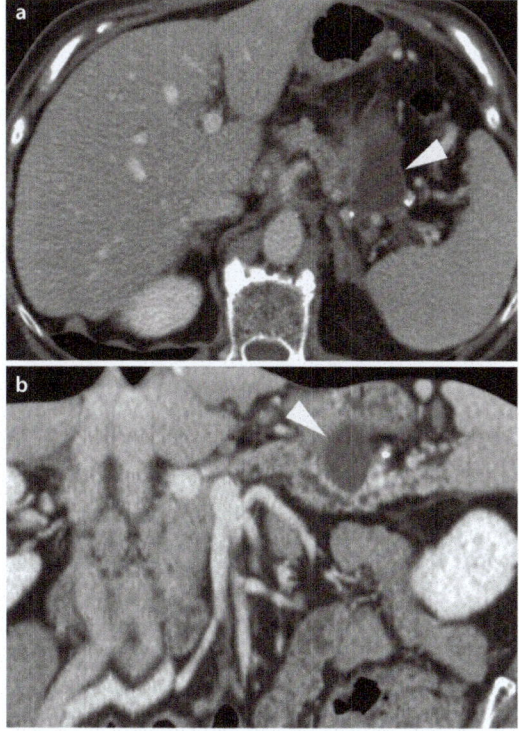

□ Fig. 8.1 Mucinous cystic adenoma of the tail of the pancreas. Female, 55 years old. Contrast-enhanced CT-scan on axial plane **a** and curvilinear reconstruction **b** show a unicystic lesion of the tail of the pancreas (*arrowhead* in **a** and **b**) without visible septations. The lesion has a thin wall, without papillary projections, and does not show any communication with the main pancreatic duct, which is dilated. Stranding of the peripancreatic fat around the lesion could mean infiltration of adjacent organs

Mucinous cystic neoplasms are large, ranging from 2 to 36 cm, with an average size of 10 cm. The tumors are round with well-defined margins; however, a bosselated or lobulated surface may be seen. Cut sections of a typical mucinous cystic neoplasm reveal a multilocular cystic lesion with thin septations measuring less than 2 mm in greatest thickness (□ Fig. 8.1). The cystic cavities vary in size and measure up to many centimeters in greatest dimension. The internal surface of the cyst may contain thin papillary projections into the lumen. In rare cases, a single dominant cystic cavity or a unilocular cystic mass may be seen. The lesions do not normally communicate with the pancreatic duct. Thickness of septa and presence of parietal nodules and papillary vegetations are correlated with malignancy [6] (□ Figs. 8.2 and 8.3).

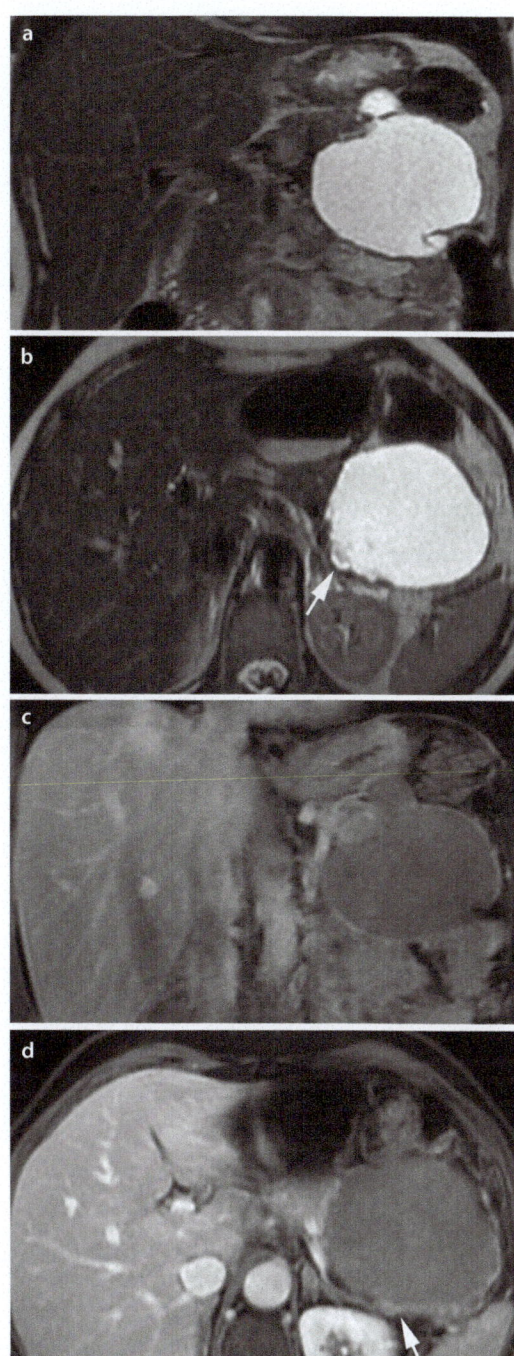

□ Fig. 8.2 Mucinous cystoadenocarcinoma. Fifty-eight-year-old woman. Coronal **a** and axial **b** T2-weighted MR images demonstrated a large cystic lesion of the tail of the pancreas with hyperintense fluid content and various papillary projections (*arrow* in **b**). Coronal **c** and axial **d** T1-weighted MR images after contrast administration show enhancement of the wall and the projections (*arrow* in **d**)

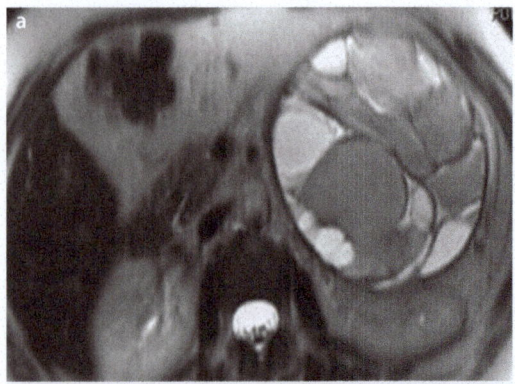

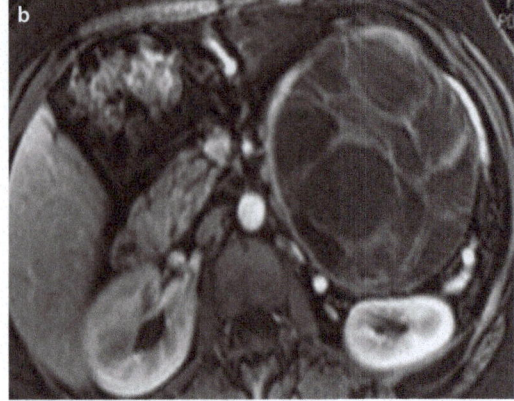

□ **Fig. 8.3** Mucinous cystic adenocarcinoma of the tail of the pancreas. Female, 48 years old. A very large multiloculated cystic mass of the tail of the pancreas is seen on axial **a** T2-weighted MR images. The content of the different cysts is hyper or isointense on T2-weighted MR images due to different mucin components. The mass shows many irregular and thick internal septations with enhancement on axial **b** T1-weighted imaged after contrast administration

Guidelines	Criteria
Sendai consensus guidelines	
High risk	Symptomatic
	Size ≥3 cm
	Solid component/mural nodules
	Dilated main duct (≥5 mm)
Fukuoka consensus guidelines	
High risk	Proximal lesion with obstructive jaundice
	Solid component/mural nodules
	Dilated main duct (≥10 mm)
Worrisome	Size ≥3 cm
	Pancreatitis
	Thickened, enhancing walls
	Dilated duct (5–10 mm)
	Change in duct caliber with distal atrophy
	Lymphadenopathy

□ **Table 8.1**   Sendai and Fukuoka criteria for risk assessment of IPMN and MCN

8.1.3 Clinical Management

Since complete surgical excision can result in good prognosis and 5-year disease-specific survival for noninvasive MCNs is 100% while for those with invasive cancer is only 57%, surgical excision and long-term follow-up are the treatment of choice for patients with MCNs. Although most patients with MCNs undergo tumor resection, the surgical indications have become considerably more conservative with the introduction of Sendai and Fukuoka consensus guidelines which defined the characteristics of high-risk neoplasms (□ Table 8.1).

8.2 Patterns of Local Spread

8.2.1 Introduction

Many studies showed that a single MCN can harbor different degrees of dysplasia, from adenoma to invasive carcinoma. The prevalence of invasive cancer is only 12%. Two degrees of invasion were defined: intracapsular, if neoplastic invasion did not go beyond the outer layer of the wall; extracapsular, if it extended into the surrounding pancreatic and extrapancreatic tissue. Only patients with invasive cancer diffusely invading into or beyond the tumor wall are at substantial risk of distant or local recurrence, whereas those with intracapsular foci of invasive carcinoma have a much better prognosis. Unfortunately, once recurrence is diagnosed, the prognosis is very poor: in the study by Crippa, all seven patients with tumor recurrence died after a mean of 6.5 months [7].

8.2.2 Vessel Infiltration

Although macroscopic vessel infiltration is not described in the literature, resectability criteria devised for adenocarcinoma can be used also for mucinous adenocarcinoma (see ▶ Chap. 6, ◘ Tables 6.5 and 6.6). Since tumor location is in 95% in the body-tail, splenic artery and vein should be the vessels more frequently involved and, unless the celiac axis is involved at the origin, tumors should be always resectable. In a recent multicenter study only microvascular infiltration was demonstrated and only in 10.5% of cases [7].

8.2.3 Lymph Node Metastases

Although no specific data with regard to node status are mentioned in the literature for MCNs defined by ovarian stroma, Crippa et al. [7] observed a complete absence of lymph node metastases in patients with invasive carcinoma, despite sampling of an average of 14 nodes in 19 patients. Interestingly, ovarian mucinous neoplasms show a similar biologic behavior, with lymph node metastases reported in less than 10% of the cases. Because the probability of malignancy is very low in patients with small MCNs without nodules, lymphadenectomy can be avoided and parenchyma-sparing procedures such as middle pancreatectomy and perhaps enucleations should be performed more often, because they decrease the rate of postoperative pancreatic insufficiency and they have been proven to be safe in the treatment of well-selected patients with MCNs.

8.2.4 Neural Infiltration

Mucinous adenocarcinoma does not show a high tendency to perineural invasion: in a recent study this was demonstrated in only 16% of cases [7]. Because of the peculiar tumor location, in case of perineural invasion the splenic plexus is the most frequent site of invasion; the second site of invasion is a direct route leading to the celiac ganglion via a distinct nerve trunk, which runs independently of blood vessels.

8.2.5 Peritoneal Dissemination

As described above, mucins in cancer cells contribute to carcinogenesis and tumor invasion by simultaneously disrupting existing interactions and establishing new ones. These tumors produce variable amounts of intracellular and/or extracellular mucins. For these reasons, the peculiar dissemination of mucinous adenocarcinoma of the pancreas is peritoneal. Pseudomixoma peritonei is a peculiar condition characterized by accumulation of copious gelatinous materials throughout the peritoneal cavity. In the literature few cases of pseudomixoma peritonei associated with pancreatic neoplasms have been reported. Peritoneal lesions can be infiltrative, micronodular or macronodular, with coexistence of different patterns of spread in a single case. Nodular lesion can present enhancement after administration of contrast material or can be hypoattenuating due to simil-cystic appearance. Sometimes they can show microcalcifications. The mesenteric scirrhotic involvement usually manifests with thickening of the roots of the sheats. In advanced cases thickening and enhancement of peritoneal reflections coexist with soft tissue nodules and stranding and thickening of the omentum (omental cake).

8.3 Intraductal Papillary Mucinous Neoplasms

8.3.1 Epidemiology

Once considered as "rare" entities, intraductal papillary mucinous neoplasms (IPMN) nowadays represent the most frequent cystic neoplasm of the pancreas even in asymptomatic patients, in which they usually constitute an incidental finding [8]. The first report of this pathology was made by Ohashi in 1982 [3], and afterwards the knowledge of this emerging disease has significantly improved so that it was included in the classification of the exocrine pancreatic neoplasms proposed by the World Health Organization (WHO) in 1996 [9].

The WHO has defined IPMNs as intraductal papillary mucinous neoplasms with tall, columnar, mucin-containing epithelium, with or without papillary projections, involving the main pancreatic duct and/or its branch ducts.

The WHO classification was updated in 2000 [10] and 2010 [11]; these updates divided the tumors in two different entities according to the site of origin: branch-duct and main-duct IPMNs that seem to have a more aggressive behavior [12, 13].

Although the real incidence of IPMNs is still unknown, it is consistently increasing in the last decades. In some surgical series, IPMN represent 8% of all pancreatic resections [14].

8

8.3.2 Pathology

According to the 2010 WHO classification, IPMNs are subdivided into two different entities: main-duct IPMNs (MD-IPMNs) and branch-duct IPMNs (BD-IPMNs). IPMNs that involve both the main pancreatic duct and the branch ducts are defined mixed IPMNs [15].

MD-IPMNs involve the main pancreatic duct and are usually located in the proximal portion of the gland (75%), but they can spread to the rest of the main pancreatic duct. They usually presents as a dilated (≥1 cm) main pancreatic duct full of mucus that may extrude through a bulging ampulla, although it can also appear as a "cyst" along the main pancreatic duct (◘ Figs. 8.4 and 8.5).

BD-IPMNs involve the side branches of the pancreatic ductal system, more commonly in the uncinate process, even if they are described in the whole gland, appearing as a cystic lesion communicating with a non-dilated main pancreatic duct.

Mixed-type IPMNs involve both the main pancreatic duct and the side branches of the ductal system (◘ Fig. 8.6).

Noninvasive intraductal papillary mucinous neoplasms are classified based on the highest degree of cytoarchitectural atypia into three categories: low-grade dysplasia, moderate dysplasia, and high-grade dysplasia/carcinoma in situ. Invasive neoplasms are classified as IPMN with an associated invasive carcinoma.

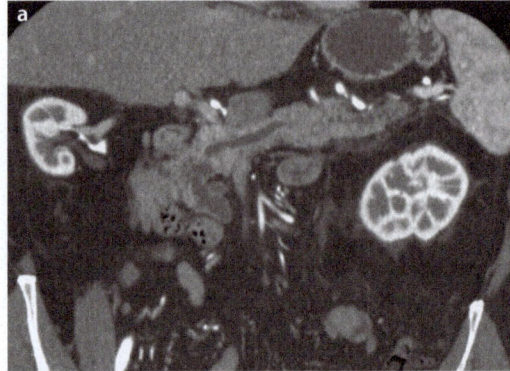
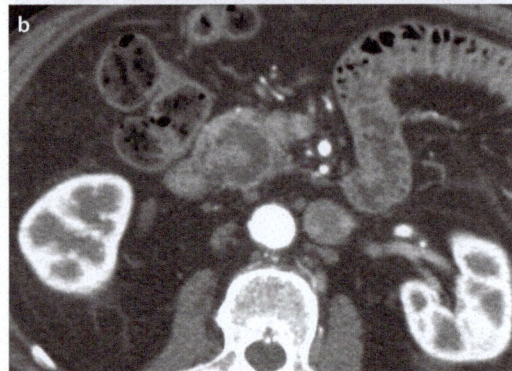
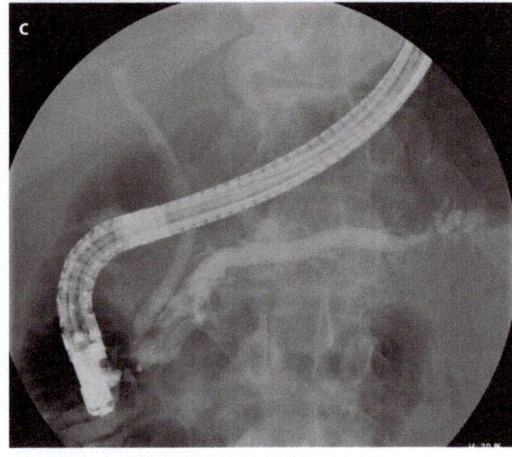

◘ **Fig. 8.4** Main-duct intraductal papillary mucinous neoplasm of the pancreas. Male, 73 years old. Contrast-enhanced portal venous phase CT-scan on curved multiplanar reconstruction **a** and axial **b** plane. The main pancreatic duct is irregularly dilated, mostly in the head of the gland. ERCP **c** shows the dilatation of the entire course of the main pancreatic duct with small parietal irregularities at the head and tail of the pancreas

Considering the epithelial subtypes, tubular, colloid, and oncocytic invasive IPMNs have varying prognoses. Colloid and oncocytic types have markedly improved biology, whereas the tubular type has a course that resembles ductal adenocarcinoma (◘ Fig. 8.7).

■ **Fig. 8.5** Main-duct intraductal papillary mucinous neoplasm. Female, 78 years old. Axial T2 weighted MR image **a** and MRCP **b** show an irregularly dilated main pancreatic duct in its entire length. No enhancing nodules or parietal thickening are visible in the arterial phase both in the axial T1-post contrast MR image **c** and in the curved-MPR CT image **d**

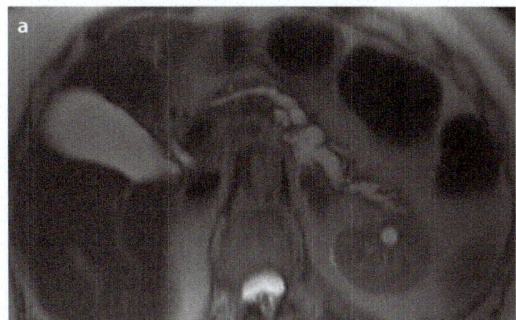

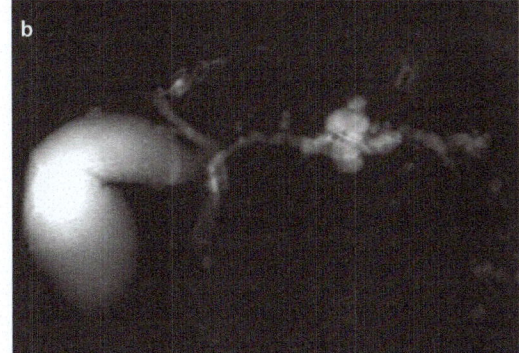

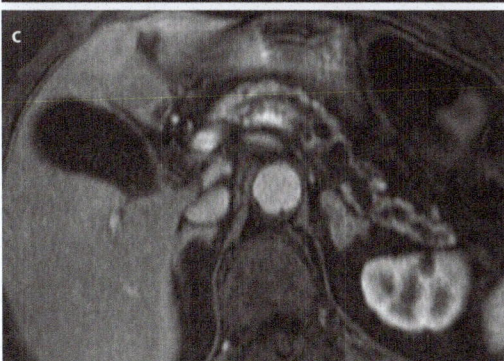

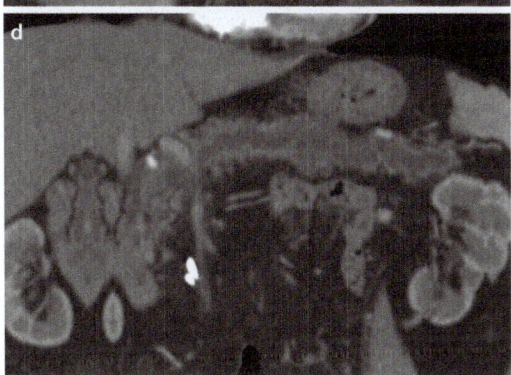

The histological subtypes of adenocarcinoma arising in the background of IPMN appear to correlate with a specific epithelial subtype. All the invasive IPMNs with colloid carcinoma originate in the background of intestinal-type IPMN, and those with oncocytic carcinoma are seen only on the background of oncocytic-type IPMN. The majority of tubular adenocarcinomas (66%) originate in gastric-type IPMNs, although rare tubular adenocarcinomas were also found to arise in the background of pancreatobiliary-type (13%), intestinal-type (16%), and oncocytic-type (5%) IPMNs [16].

The histology of invasive components has also been associated with the type of duct involvement by IPMN. It has been described that main-duct-type IPMNs often exhibit intestinal-type epithelium, and branch-duct-type IPMNs usually show gastric-type epithelium [17].

8.3.3 Clinical Management

While the management of BD-IPMN has undergone modifications over time, the treatment of MD-IPMN has not changed much over the past three decades. Most patients with MD-IPMN who are fit for surgery undergo tumor resection. On the contrary, the surgical indications for branch-duct-type IPMN (BD-IPMN) have become considerably more conservative. The Sendai guidelines published in 2006 proposed a variety of strategies for the management of IPMN (■ Table 8.1) [5]. The guidelines recommended resection of most BD-IPMN measuring >3 cm in diameter even without mural nodules, and many patients with these tumors therefore underwent resection. As malignancy was found in 25.5% of all resected BD-IPMNs and invasive cancer was found in 17.7%, the later Fukuoka guidelines included more conservative criteria for the surgical resection of BD-IPMN [18]. They adopt two layers of criteria for assessment of IPMN: "*high-risk stigmata*" considered to be indicative of malignancy, and "*worrisome features*" possibly pointing towards malignancy. The high-risk stigmata include obstructive jaundice, enhancing solid component, and main pancreatic duct size ≥10 mm: patients with these features should undergo resection without delay. The worrisome features include a cyst size ≥3 cm, thickened and enhancing cyst walls, non-enhancing mural

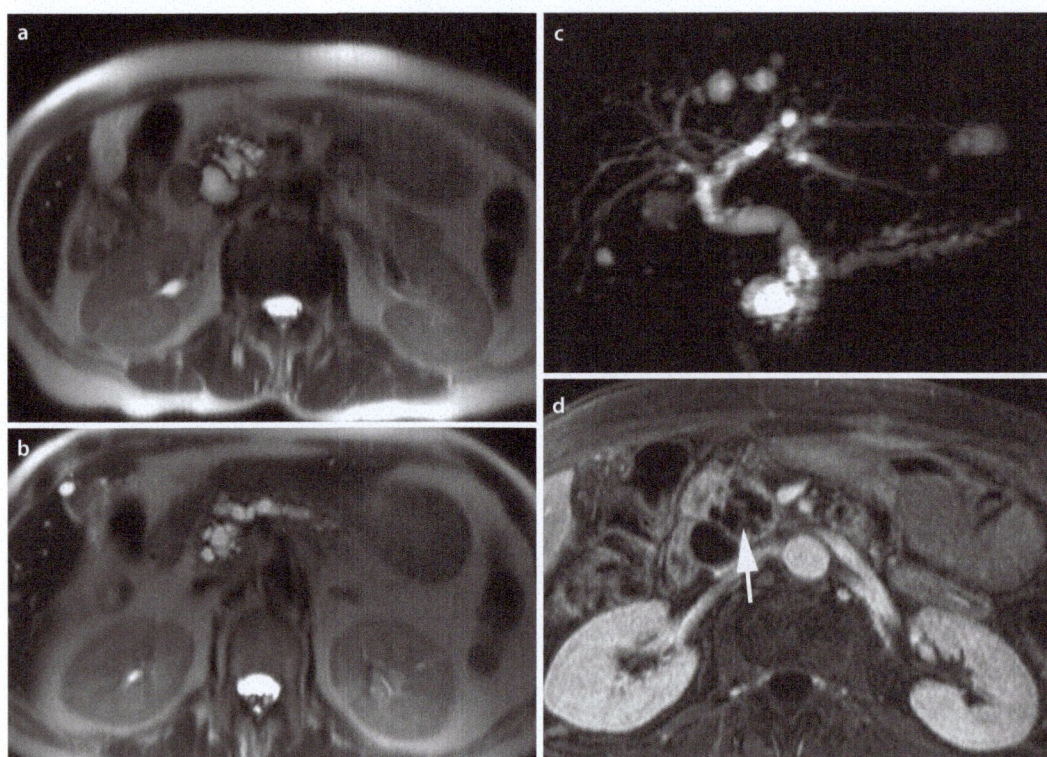

Fig. 8.6 Mixed-type intraductal papillary mucinous neoplasm. Female, 68 years old. Axial T2-weighted MR images **a**, **b** and MRCP **c** show marked dilatation of the main pancreatic duct and branch ducts of the whole gland. Some papillary vegetations which show enhancement in axial T1-weighted portal venous phase (*arrow* in **d**) are visible inside the ducts of the head of the pancreas

nodules, main pancreatic duct size 5–9 mm, an abrupt change in the main pancreatic duct caliber with distal pancreatic atrophy, and lymphadenopathy on imaging examinations; and clinical acute pancreatitis. Patients with these features should be evaluated by endoscopic ultrasonography (EUS) for further risk stratification. The use of these two layers of criteria seems to result in more accurate assessment of the need for surgical treatment of BD-IPMN [19].

8.4 Patterns of Local Spread

8.4.1 Invasive Cancer and IPMN

Invasive cancers arising from IPMNs are recognized as a morphologically and biologically heterogeneous group of neoplasms. Considering all ductal types, the proportion of invasive IPMC among total IPMN ranges from 19 to 50%, and the 5-year survival rate of invasive IPMN is reported to range from 31 to 78% [20].

On the other hand, PDAC with an associated IPMN represents another extreme of invasive IPMC. Pancreatic ductal adenocarcinoma located in the environs of IPMN makes it difficult to distinguish whether the IPMN is the precursor or a coincident condition of PDAC. However, both PDAC derived from IPMN and PDAC concomitant with IPMN revealed better prognostic outcome compared with conventional PDAC.

Some authors indicate that concomitant pancreatic cancer occurs in 2–10% of patients with IPMN [21–29]. Even a small (≤1 cm diameter) BD-IPMN is associated with an 8% risk of developing distinct pancreatic cancer during surveillance [22]. The reported yearly incidence of distinct pancreatic cancer in patients with BD-IPMN is 0.41–1.10% [22, 24, 28].

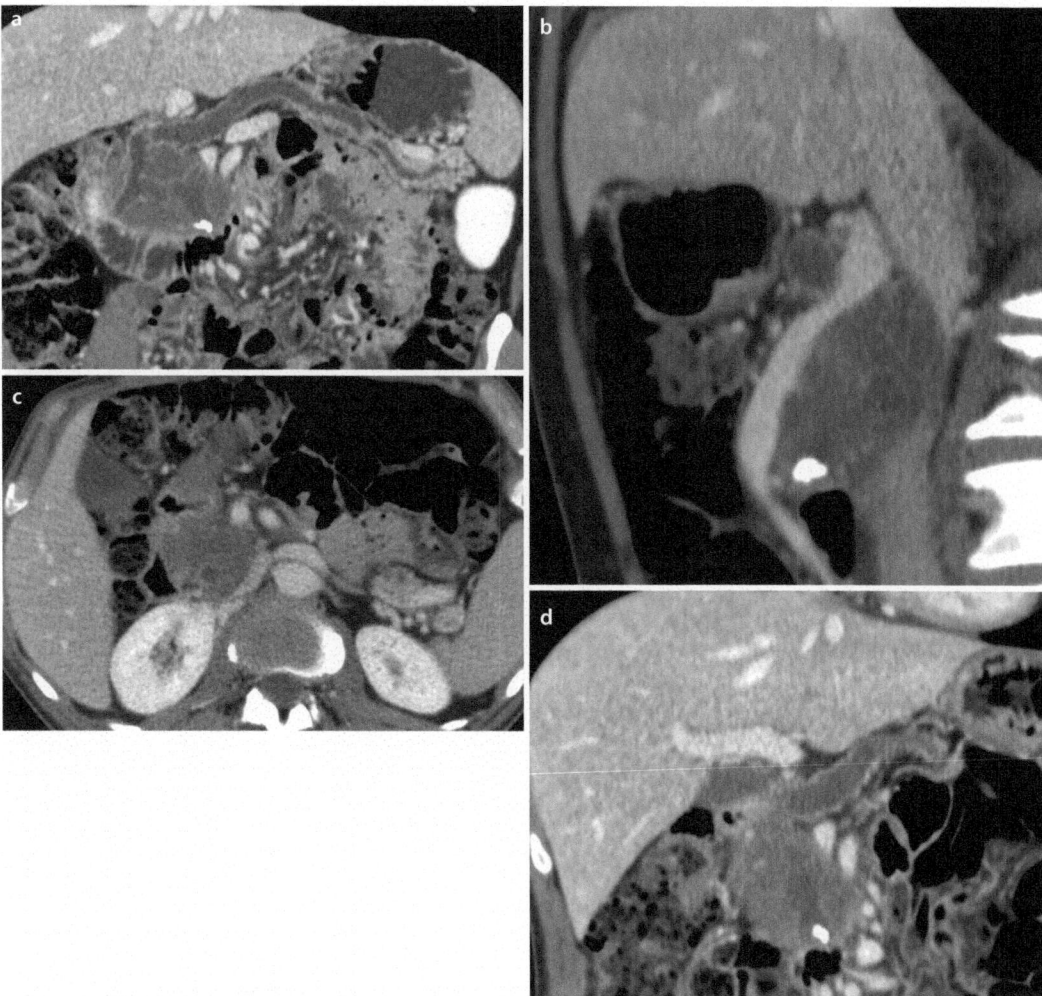

◻ Fig. 8.7 Intraductal papillary mucinous neoplasm with associated invasive colloid-type adenocarcinoma. Fifty-seven-year-old male. Contrast-enhanced MDCT on coronal **a, d**, sagittal **b**, and axial **c** planes shows a large hypovascular mass of the head of the pancreas without fat cleavage planes with the duodenal wall and with encasement of the superior mesenteric vein. The main pancreatic duct is well visible, dilated in the whole gland with atrophy of the parenchyma in the body of the pancreas

Invasive IPMN, as a whole, appears to have improved survival compared with pancreatic ductal adenocarcinoma (PDAC), but there are conflicting results as to whether the improved survival of invasive IPMN is confirmed when the tumors are matched by stage.

8.4.2 Vessel Infiltration

As for pancreatic adenocarcinoma, the arterial pattern of encasement is defined as obliteration of the fat plane of less than 50% or obliteration of at least 50% for the celiac trunk and the hepatic and superior mesenteric arteries. Venous pattern of encasement is defined as complete circumferential obliteration of the fat plane of 50% or more, deformation of the superior mesenteric vein into the tear drop sign, or thrombosis or obliteration of the lumen. Obliteration of the fat plane for less than 50% is not considered venous encasement. Although no other different criteria of resectability for vessel infiltration have been proposed yet, some authors observed that vascular criteria are less accurate in the evaluation of resectability of IPMN than in the case of pancreatic carcinoma. In a recent study, the overall accuracy of helical CT in determining surgical resectability of malignant IPMNs when using adenocarcinoma criteria was 74%, the positive predictive value in determining whether malignant IPMNs were resectable was 100% while the positive predictive value of helical CT in determining whether malignant IPMNs were unresectable was only 17% [30]. This was likely due to the common peripancreatic inflammatory changes that occur in these patients secondary to pancreatitis (which occurs in 30% of patients with IPMN and 3% of patients with adenocarcinoma), resulting in peripancreatic fat stranding mimicking carcinomatosis on CT.

8.4.3 Lymph Node Involvement

Considering that the sequence of lymph node involvement is the same of pancreatic adenocarcinoma, according to the different location of the tumor, lymph node involvement occurs less frequently in patients with IPMN than in those with adenocarcinoma. In a recent study, lymph node involvement was found in 25% of patients with IPMN, including 58% of those with invasive tumors, and in 76% of patients with adenocarcinoma [30].

8.4.4 Neural Infiltration

Although, depending on the tumor site, the pattern of neural invasion is comparable to that of PDAC, some studies reported a lower perineural invasion rate for invasive IPMN when compared to PDAC (49.2% vs. 76.5%) [31]. When present it is associated with unfavorable long-term outcome [32].

8.4.5 Peritoneal Dissemination

As already described for mucinous adenocarcinoma, in tumors producing intracellular or extracellular mucins cancer cells carcinogenesis and tumor spread can occur with peritoneal dissemination (◘ Figs. 8.8 and 8.9). Since IPMN are

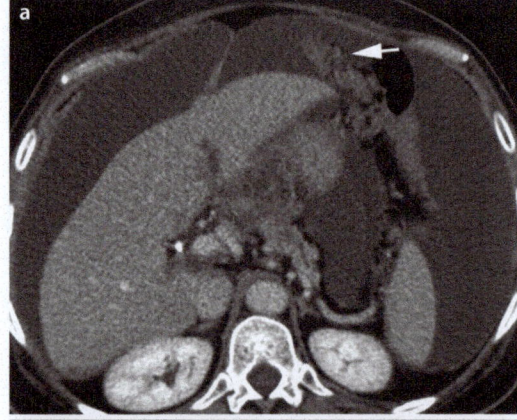
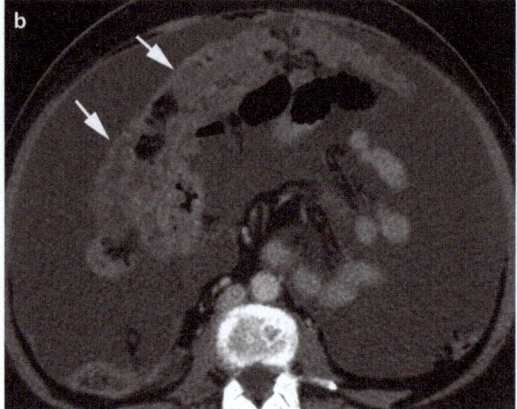

◘ **Fig. 8.8** Intraductal papillary neoplasm associated with ductal adenocarcinoma of the pancreas. Female, 61 years old. Contrast-enhanced portal venous phase CT-scan axial plane **a, b**. At the head of the pancreas a mixed lesion, with predominantly cystic component and irregularly thickened walls and septa is well depicted. The main pancreatic duct at the body and tail of the pancreas is slightly dilated. Pseudomixoma peritonei is well visible with peritoneal reflections, soft tissue nodules, and stranding of the omentum (omental cake, *arrow*)

characterized by intraductal proliferation of mucinous epithelia growing within cystically dilated pancreatic ducts, pseudomixoma peritonei can be their initial clinical presentation or sign of recurrence [33]. As already specified pseudomixoma peritonei is characterized by accumulation of copious gelatinous materials throughout the peritoneal cavity. Only few cases of IPMN with pseudomixoma peritonei have been reported in which the causes where iatrogenic (by surgical intervention or by endosonographically guided fine-needle aspiration biopsy) or a latent rupture or fistula formation of the IPMN into the peritoneal cavity [33–35].

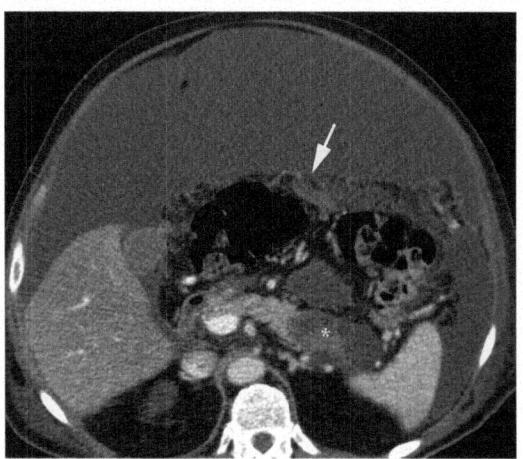

◘ Fig. 8.9 Invasive intraductal papillary neoplasm of the pancreas. Male, 68 years old. Contrast-enhanced portal venous phase CT on axial plane. A heterogeneous lesion of the tail of the pancreas is depicted. The lesion has a solid (*asterisk* in **a**) and cystic components and shows communication with the main pancreatic duct. Pseudomixoma peritonei is well visible with peritoneal reflections, soft tissue nodules, and stranding of the omentum (omental cake, *arrow*)

References

1. Rosenberger LH et al (2012) Intraductal papillary mucinous neoplasm (IPMN) with extra-pancreatic mucin: a case series and review of the literature. J Gastrointest Surg 16(4):762–770
2. Compagno J, Oertel JE (1978) Mucinous cystic neoplasms of the pancreas with overt and latent malignancy (cystadenocarcinoma and cystadenoma). A clinicopathologic study of 41 cases. Am J Clin Pathol 69(6):573–580
3. Ohashi K (1982) Four cases of mucus secreting pancreatic cancer. Prog Dig Endoscopy 20:348–351
4. Buetow PC, Rao P, Thompson LD (1998) From the archives of the AFIP. Mucinous cystic neoplasms of the pancreas: radiologic-pathologic correlation. Radiographics 18(2):433–449
5. Tanaka M et al (2006) International consensus guidelines for management of intraductal papillary mucinous neoplasms and mucinous cystic neoplasms of the pancreas. Pancreatology 6(1–2):17–32
6. Procacci C et al (2001) CT features of malignant mucinous cystic tumors of the pancreas. Eur Radiol 11(9):1626–1630
7. Crippa S et al (2008) Mucinous cystic neoplasm of the pancreas is not an aggressive entity: lessons from 163 resected patients. Ann Surg 247(4):571–579
8. Carbognin G et al (2006) Branch duct IPMTs: value of cross-sectional imaging in the assessment of biological behavior and follow-up. Abdom Imaging 31(3):320–325
9. Kloppel G, Solci E, Capella C, Longnecker DS (1996) Histological typing of tumours of the exocrine pancreas. World Health Organization international histological classification of tumours. Springer, Berlin
10. Longnecker DS, Adler G, Hruban RH, Kloppel G (2000) Intraductal papillary-mucinous neoplasms of the pancreas. In: WHO classification of tumors of the digestive system, p 23–40
11. Bosman FT CF, Hruban RH, Theise ND (2010) WHO classification of tumors of digestive system. In: Adsay FN NV, Furukawa T, Huruban RH, Klimstra DS, Kloppel G (eds) Intraductal neoplasm of the pancreas, 4th edn. Lyon
12. Kobari M et al (1999) Intraductal papillary mucinous tumors of the pancreas comprise 2 clinical subtypes: differences in clinical characteristics and surgical management. Arch Surg 134(10):1131–1136
13. Terris B et al (2000) Intraductal papillary mucinous tumors of the pancreas confined to secondary ducts show less aggressive pathologic features as compared with those involving the main pancreatic duct. Am J Surg Pathol 24(10):1372–1377
14. Fernandez-del Castillo C, Adsay NV (2010) Intraductal papillary mucinous neoplasms of the pancreas. Gastroenterology 139(3):708–13, 713.e1–2
15. Procacci C et al (2001) Intraductal papillary mucinous tumors of the pancreas: spectrum of CT and MR findings with pathologic correlation. Eur Radiol 11(10): 1939–1951
16. Mino-Kenudson M et al (2011) Prognosis of invasive intraductal papillary mucinous neoplasm depends on histological and precursor epithelial subtypes. Gut 60(12):1712–1720
17. Furukawa T et al (2011) Prognostic relevance of morphological types of intraductal papillary mucinous neoplasms of the pancreas. Gut 60(4):509–516
18. Tanaka M et al (2012) International consensus guidelines 2012 for the management of IPMN and MCN of the pancreas. Pancreatology 12(3):183–197
19. Ohno E et al (2009) Intraductal papillary mucinous neoplasms of the pancreas: differentiation of malignant and benign tumors by endoscopic ultrasound findings of mural nodules. Ann Surg 249(4):628–634
20. Kang MJ et al (2013) Disease spectrum of intraductal papillary mucinous neoplasm with an associated invasive carcinoma invasive IPMN versus pancreatic ductal adenocarcinoma-associated IPMN. Pancreas 42(8):1267–1274
21. Tada M et al (2006) Pancreatic cancer in patients with pancreatic cystic lesions: a prospective study in 197 patients. Clin Gastroenterol Hepatol 4(10):1265–1270
22. Uehara H et al (2008) Development of ductal carcinoma of the pancreas during follow-up of branch duct intraductal papillary mucinous neoplasm of the pancreas. Gut 57(11):1561–1565
23. Ingkakul T et al (2010) Predictors of the presence of concomitant invasive ductal carcinoma in intraductal papillary mucinous neoplasm of the pancreas. Ann Surg 251(1):70–75
24. Tanno S et al (2010) Pancreatic ductal adenocarcinomas in long-term follow-up patients with branch duct intraductal papillary mucinous neoplasms. Pancreas 39(1):36–40
25. Tanno S et al (2010) Incidence of synchronous and metachronous pancreatic carcinoma in 168 patients with branch duct intraductal papillary mucinous neoplasm. Pancreatology 10(2–3):173–178

26. Ikeuchi N et al (2010) Prognosis of cancer with branch duct type IPMN of the pancreas. World J Gastroenterol 16(15):1890–1895

27. Kanno A et al (2010) Prediction of invasive carcinoma in branch type intraductal papillary mucinous neoplasms of the pancreas. J Gastroenterol 45(9):952–959

28. Maguchi H et al (2011) Natural history of branch duct intraductal papillary mucinous neoplasms of the pancreas: a multicenter study in Japan. Pancreas 40(3):364–370

29. Tanaka M (2011) Controversies in the management of pancreatic IPMN. Nat Rev Gastroenterol Hepatol 8(1):56–60

30. Vullierme MP et al (2007) Malignant intraductal papillary mucinous neoplasm of the pancreas: in situ versus invasive carcinoma surgical resectability. Radiology 245(2):483–490

31. Koh YX et al (2014) Systematic review and meta-analysis comparing the surgical outcomes of invasive intraductal papillary mucinous neoplasms and conventional pancreatic ductal adenocarcinoma. Ann Surg Oncol 21(8):2782–2800

32. Marsoner K et al (2016) Pancreatic resection for intraductal papillary mucinous neoplasm- a thirteen-year single center experience. BMC Cancer 16(1):844

33. Jhuang JY, Hsieh MS (2012) Pseudomyxoma peritonei (mucinous carcinoma peritonei) preceded by intraductal papillary neoplasm of the bile duct. Hum Pathol 43(7):1148–1152

34. Mizuta Y et al (2005) Pseudomyxoma peritonei accompanied by intraductal papillary mucinous neoplasm of the pancreas. Pancreatology 5(4–5):470–474

35. Lee SE et al (2007) Intraductal papillary mucinous carcinoma with atypical manifestations: report of two cases. World J Gastroenterol 13(10):1622–1625

8

The manufacturer's authorised representative in the EU is Springer
Nature Customer Service Centre GmbH, Europaplatz 3, 69115 Heidelberg,
Germany. If you have any concerns regarding our products, please
contact ProductSafety@springernature.com

Printed and bound by CPI Group (UK) Ltd, Croydon, CR0 4YY
29/04/2026
02099451-0020